How to be a Laboratory Biosafety Officer third edition
by Philip A. Dauterman, MD
Table of Contents

I0494491

Chapter 1 – Introduction to lab biosafety and biosecurity

In its strictest definition, laboratory biosafety refers to the practices and procedures used to handle infectious specimens, cultures of organisms and potentially infectious waste. The purpose is to prevent laboratory acquired infections (LAI) and/or contamination of the environment.

The job of a Laboratory Biosafety Officer (BSO) has been expanded to include virtually all aspects of safety in the clinical laboratory. The job description of the typical Lab BSO is:

1. educates and trains everyone in lab (lab staff, visitors, contractors, etc.) on lab biosafety.
2. performs risk assessments of the lab and mitigates the risks.
3. receives reports of safety issues, and works to correct any issues identified.
4. writes biosafety policies and procedures including a Biosafety Manual.
5. enforces the biosafety policies, rules and regulations on everyone in lab.
6. responsible for safe shipping of hazardous material to and from the laboratory.
7. available on-call 24 hours a day, 7 days a week as needed for emergencies, spills, etc.
8. prepares reports for the hospital-wide safety committee.
9. ensures compliance with all biosafety related regulatory requirements.
10. provides technical advice as needed to the lab staff, Lab Supervisor, Lab Director and/or Medical Staff.
11. provides leadership to the lab staff.
12. must have outstanding communication skills.
13. may be required to provide outreach. Outreach refers to working outside your own organization to assist outside organizations with their own biosafety and biosecurity. For example, a one-day assignment to a Public Health facility outside your usual work organization to evaluate their biocontainment, preparedness, etc.
14. other duties as assigned.

The above list of duties is "all hazard" meaning that the Lab Biosafety Officer is responsible for the physical, chemical and radiological hazard plans as well as the biological hazard plans. The typical clinical lab does not have a radiological materials permit and does not test patient samples or environmental materials for radioactivity. Only the hospital radiology department has a radiologic materials permit. Thus, the typical Lab Biosafety Officer only has to deal with physical, biological and chemical hazards. I will spend the rest of this book discussing physical, chemical and biological hazards, and will not discuss radiological hazards further.

Laboratory biosecurity is defined as measures to prevent unauthorized access to infectious materials. In the simplest terms biosafety is keeping bad organisms away from people; and biosecurity is keeping bad people away from organisms.

Chapter 2 – How to read a National Fire Protection Association (NFPA) sign

The National Fire Protection Association (NFPA) is a trade association that sets standards for fire codes. NFPA standard 704 is a system of signage used to identify chemical hazards. This signage is not used for biologic or other hazards. It is referred to as the "fire diamond" due to its diamond shape. Clockwise from top, the red diamond stands for flammability, the yellow diamond stands for reactivity, the white diamond stands for other considerations and the blue diamond stands for health hazards. An example is given on the next page.

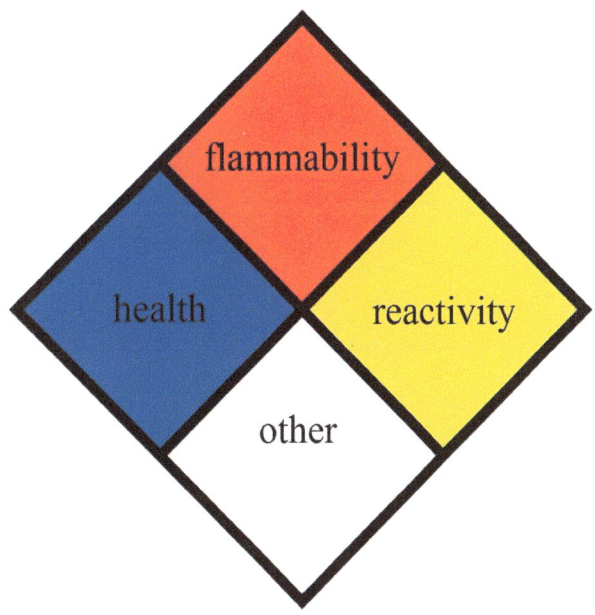

The red, yellow and blue diamonds are rated from 0 to 4 as follows:

Red diamond = flammability

0. will not burn
1. requires heating over 93.3 °C (200 °F) to ignite
2. requires heating between 37.8° and 93.3 °C (100° and 200 °F) to ignite
3. ignites around room temperature
4. ignites below room temperature

Yellow diamond = reactivity

0. stable even in fires
1. stable except in fires
2. reacts violently in fires or water
3. capable of explosion but requires significant heating
4. explosive at room temperature

Blue Diamond = health hazard

0. nontoxic
1. causes minor irritation
2. causes intense irritation to minor incapacitation
3. short exposure could cause permanent injury
4. very short exposure could be fatal

White diamond = other considerations. There are only three official (and several unofficial, nonstandard) choices for this box. Most often the white diamond will be left blank. The three official symbols that can be put in are:

OX = Oxidizer
W̶ = Reacts with water (do not use water based fire extinguishers)
SA = Simple asphyxiant gas

Let me give as an example the NFPA sign for 100% ethanol:

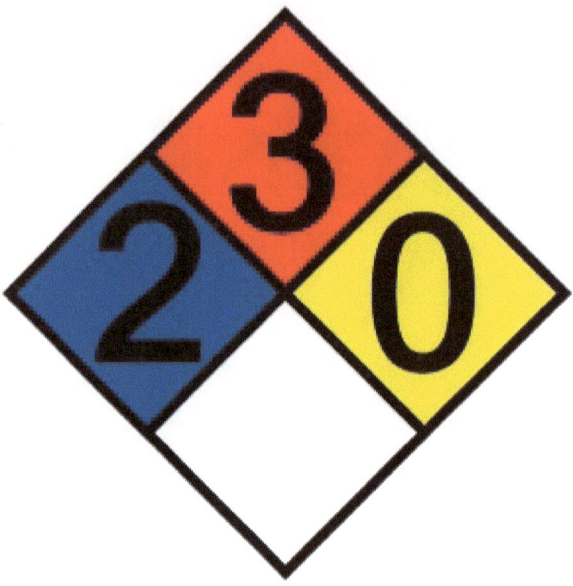

The above sign indicates 100% ethanol has a flammability of 3 (ignites around room temperature) a health hazard of 2 (causes intense irritation to minor incapacitation) and a reactivity of 0 (stable).

As another example, here is the NFPA sign for hydrochloric acid:

The above sign indicates that hydrochloric acid has a flammability of 0 (will not burn) a health hazard of 3 (short exposure could cause permanent injury) and a reactivity of 1 (stable except in fires).

If you have multiple different chemicals in storage in the same fire cabinet, the NFPA sign on the front of the fire cabinet should include the highest number for each of the numbered diamonds. For example, if you have both hydrochloric acid and 100% ethanol in the same fire cabinet, the NFPA sign should be as follows:

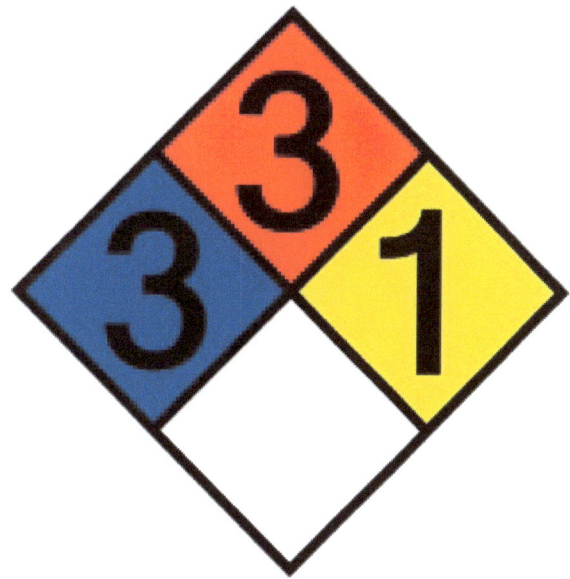

The red diamond representing flammability is set at 3 due to 100% ethanol's flammability rating of 3. Ethanol's flammability of 3 is higher than hydrochloric acid's flammability of 0; therefore the 3 from ethanol goes on the sign on the front of the fire cabinet. The yellow diamond representing reactivity is set a 1 due to hydrochloric acid's reactivity of 1. The blue diamond representing health hazard is set at 3 due to hydrochloric acid's health hazard of 3. The white diamond is left blank since there is nothing in the white diamond for either 100% ethanol or hydrochloric acid.

If your fire cabinet has large numbers of different chemicals in it, you will need to sort through to see which has the highest flammability, which has the highest reactivity, etc. You will need to set the diamonds of the NFPA fire symbol to match the highest number for flammability, reactivity and health hazard of the various chemicals in the fire cabinet. The sign on the front of the fire cabinet has to match what is inside, and the contents of the cabinet have to match the sign.

As a caveat, the NFPA signs should be printed in color. My lab was cited in a recent inspection for NFPA signs printed in black-and-white. I tried to explain to the inspector that my lab did not have a color printer, and color printing is not needed since you can deduce the color of the diamond from the position of the diamond. The inspector still cited my lab and we had to get color printed NFPA signs.

Chapter 3 – How to read Globally Harmonized Pictograms

The Globally Harmonized Pictograms are another way of labeling the hazards for chemicals. These are only used for chemical hazards, not biologic or radiologic hazards. These symbols became mandatory in the US in 2015. Prior to 2015 they had only been required internationally, not is the US. The problem is that older Safety Data Sheets (SDS) in the US do not have these pictograms. My lab was cited for outdated SDS in an inspection and had to replace all our SDS with ones that had the globally harmonized pictograms. These pictograms are:

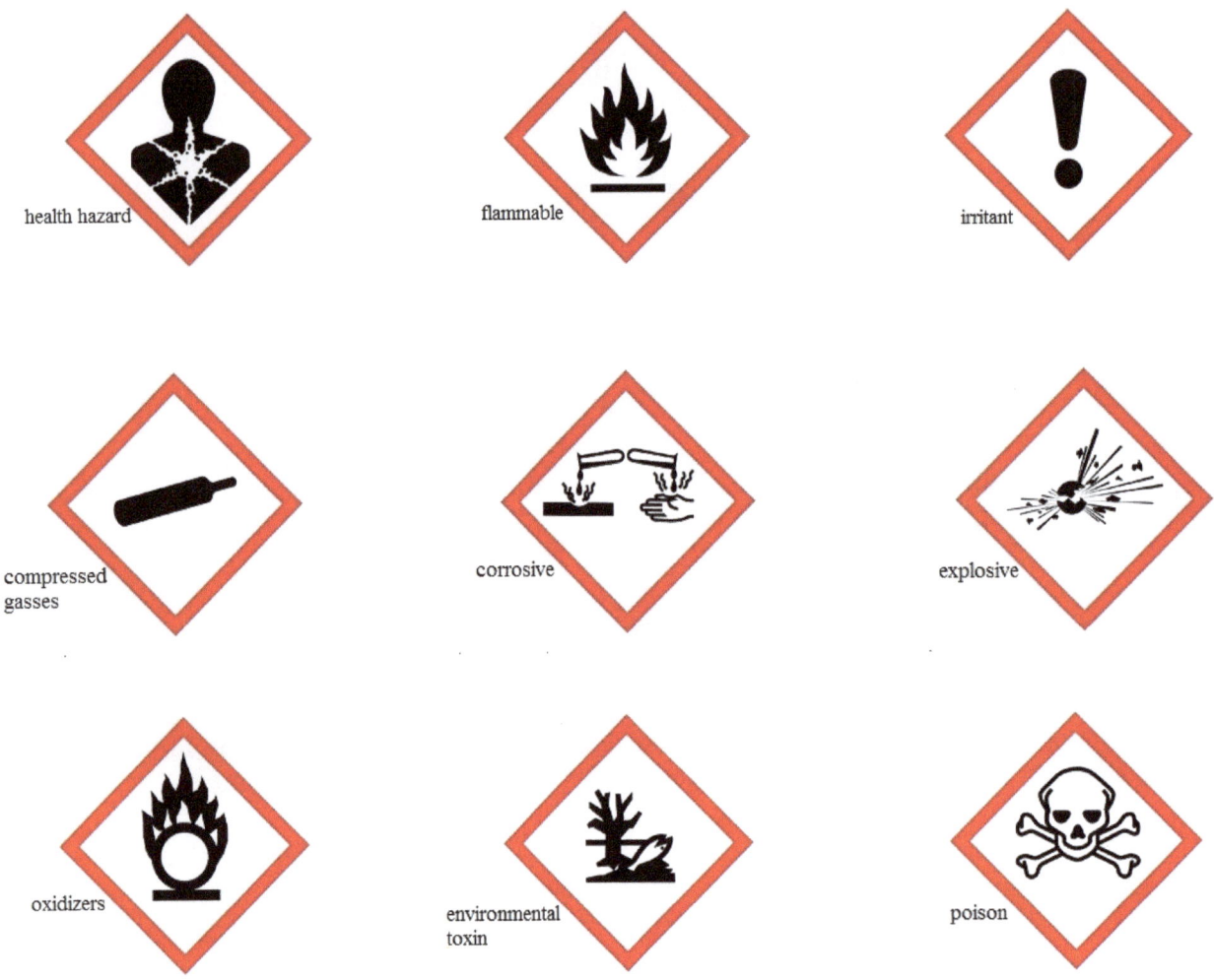

Some chemicals do not require any of these signs. For example, sodium bicarbonate does not have any of the properties listed above. Thus, the SDS for sodium bicarbonate does not contain any of the globally harmonized pictograms listed above.

Chapter 4 – Personal protective equipment, isolation precautions and infection control

The typical list of Personal Protective Equipment (PPE) found in the hospital and public health setting are:

1. Gloves
2. Gowns, aprons and lab coats
3. Masks and respirators including N95 respirators
4. Goggles and face shields
5. Shoe covers
6. The full body suit and Powered Air Purifying Respirator (PAPR) were recent additions to this list. Most hospital and public health labs got their first full body suit and PAPR at the time of the 2014 Ebola outbreak.

Some of the above list require training and/or fit testing. Hypoallergenic gloves should be available for anyone with a latex allergy. The full body suit and PAPR require training in donning and doffing, and may require fit testing. There are multiple different techniques for donning and doffing each PPE item such as gloves, gowns, face shields, etc. Multiple different institutions have pictorial diagrams of their recommended PPE donning and doffing steps available for download on the internet. In my experience PPE training is typically carried out by the hospital's Infection Control Office or Employee Health Office, and not by lab. I will not include any of the multiple different techniques for PPE donning and doffing in this book, as this training is not typically done in lab.

Some of the above list are disposable and some are reusable. Make sure the lab staff never reuse disposable PPE such as disposable gloves. Make sure that the reusable PPE such as PAPR's are being disinfected to at least the manufacturer's specifications between use. For some PPE such as lab coats not visibly soiled, the policy (disposable or reusable) can vary from one institution to another. The institutional policy has to meet or exceed the manufacturer's instructions, and cannot be less than the manufacturer's instructions. In other words the institution can have a policy to dispose of reusable lab coats after each use. However, the institution cannot have a policy to reuse gloves that the manufacturer has determined to be disposable and single use. As lab BSO, it is your responsibility to know which PPE are disposable and which PPE are reusable at your institution.

As lab BSO it is your responsibility to observe the lab staff in their use of PPE so as to ensure they are using the PPE correctly. This includes selecting the right PPE for the task at hand, checking the PPE for holes, tears, defects, etc., proper donning, all PPE donned and checked before beginning work, proper doffing, etc. As mentioned above there are numerous different techniques for donning and doffing. Do not assume the technique you learned in training is the only correct technique and all other techniques are wrong. At a minimum ensure that donning results in properly situated PPE (no gaps between gloves and lab coat sleeves, etc) and doffing is done in such a way as to avoid contamination of the user.

The Occupational Safety and Health Administration (OSHA) requires fit testing for use of the N95 respirator. The fit testing must be performed initially on employment and repeated annually and whenever the employee has physical changes that would affect the respirator fit (significant weight loss/gain, facial scarring, dental surgery, etc.). The reference is 29 CFR § 1910.134.

The N95 fit testing is not usually done in laboratory. In most hospitals the N95 fit testing is done in the Employee Health Office since the fit testing requires a medical evaluation, medical clearance and specialized equipment for the test. After completing the fit testing, the Employee Health Office will typically give the employee documentation of the fit testing. The employee will then present these papers to lab. Your lab should have documented current N95 respirator fit testing for all lab staff.

Lab staff should know which PPE to use for which task. This should be considered a basic part of orientation of new lab staff. Any prospective lab staff member should not be allowed to work independently until they have demonstrated proficiency and knowledge in the use of PPE.

New lab staff orientation is typically delegated to the section supervisor of the area where the staff will be working. If the new hire has problems with the use of PPE, understanding which PPE to use for which task, donning and doffing of PPE, etc. you as Lab Biosafety Officer may be called in to provide more training, education, supervision, and evaluation of the new staff. As Lab Biosafety Officer it is imperative that you should not allow new staff to work unsupervised if they don't show proficiency in use of PPE. Untrained or improperly trained lab staff are a disaster waiting to happen, and should be avoided at all cost.

Existing lab staff should already be trained and proficient in the use of PPE. For the existing lab staff, you will be acting as the watchdog, constantly watching the lab staff to ensure their compliance with the rules of PPE. Each lab staff is required to have competency assessment at least semiannually in the first year of employment and annually thereafter. This competency assessment is usually done by the section supervisors or Lab Supervisor. As Lab BSO, ensure that proper use of PPE is included in the competency assessment.

The various types of isolation precautions are:

1. standard precautions
2. airborne precautions
3. droplet precautions
4. contact precautions
5. protective isolation (formerly called "reverse isolation")

The phlebotomy staff that draw patients will need to be familiar with all types of precautions. The lab staff performing testing only, and not drawing patients, will only need to know standard precautions and airborne precautions.

Standard precautions, formerly called universal precautions, are used for all patients and testing. This assumes all patients have potentially infectious blood and body fluids. For lab staff this requires the use of a lab coat and gloves when drawing patients and handling specimens.

Airborne precautions are used when dealing with a potential respiratory pathogen such as tuberculosis. In addition to the standard precautions PPE, the use of an N95 or higher (i.e. N99, N100) respirator is required. For these types of lab specimens special containment is required when manipulating the specimen. See the chapter on lab biosafety containment levels.

Droplet precautions – generally only a concern for the phlebotomists drawing the patient and not for the lab staff handling the specimen. In addition to the standard precautions, add a surgical mask when entering the patient's room.

Contact precautions - generally only a concern for the phlebotomists drawing the patient and not for the lab staff handling the specimen. In addition to the standard precautions, add a disposable surgical gown when entering the patient's room. On exiting the patient's room, the surgical gown is doffed and disposed in the contaminated trash immediately and the handwashing should be especially thorough.

Protective isolation (formerly called "reverse isolation") is used for immunocompromised patients at increased risk of infection. For example, patients with very severe neutropenia must be protected from acquiring infections since they are at a higher risk of bad outcome compared to a person with a normal immune system. The types of PPE to use vary depending on the cause and severity of the patient's immunosuppression. The instructions for entry should be posted on the front door of the patient's room.

Infection control is aimed at preventing healthcare associated (i.e. nosocomial) infection. Infection control in lab includes the phlebotomist hand hygiene (handwashing or use of alcohol based hand rub) and proper use of Personal Protective Equipment (PPE) when going from patient to patient drawing blood.

Training on handwashing techniques is typically done by the hospital's Infection Control Office, and not lab. There are a multitude of different techniques for handwashing presented in the medical literature. Some require hand washing to take at least 15 seconds, others require a minimum of 20 seconds or even 30 seconds. There does not appear to be any standardization and I will not present the multitude of different techniques here. The requirements for when to perform hand hygiene seem more standardized. At a minimum hand hygiene should be performed before touching a patient, before a procedure, after a procedure, after touching a patient and after touching anything in the patient's surroundings.

The typical hospital has Infection Control observers at each nursing station. This is typically a nurse assigned the added duties of watching to make sure everyone is doffing their PPE correctly when exiting each patient's room, performing hand hygiene, and donning clean PPE when entering the next patient's room. If this observer sees anyone from lab not following the infection control policies, the observer will report the incident typically to the Infection Control Officer who will then report this to the Lab Supervisor. The Lab Supervisor is charged with enforcing all policies on the lab staff including infection control. You as Lab Biosafety Officer will likely also be notified of the occurrence.

The typical instance involves lab staff forgetting the hand hygiene between patient contacts. This is typically seen as a minor offense and typically only warrants verbal correction from the Lab Supervisor. If the same employee is reported multiple times in a short period for failure of hand hygiene, this will be taken more seriously. The employee will likely have written corrective action. You as Lab Biosafety Officer will likely be called in at this point to provide more supervision and/or corrective action to the employee in question.

In my capacity as a Lab BSO, I receive reports of lab staff failing to wash hands maybe once in three months. These reports have been for different people, not the same person every time. Everyone is human and will eventually forget to wash their hands between patient contacts. Each time this happens, I remind all the lab staff of the requirement for hand hygiene. I try not to single out the one person who forgot this time, as all will eventually forget if given enough time.

I have not seen more serious violations of Infection Control policy. If this were to occur I would call a meeting with the Infection Control Officer and the Lab Supervisor to discuss the situation and how to deal with the employee involved.

Chapter 5 – Chemical hazard containment and decontamination

The typical small hospital or public health laboratory will have a small amount of dangerous chemicals such as potassium hydroxide (used for KOH preps). Most such labs will also have small amounts of flammables (typically ethanol or other alcohols used as solvents in staining solutions). The majority of chemicals used in lab are not very toxic or flammable.

If your lab is using dangerous chemicals, these will need to be stored in a fire and/or corrosives cabinet while not in use. OSHA gives the specifications for fire cabinets at 29 CFR § 1910.106. To briefly summarize, any flammable liquid must be stored in a fire-resistant cabinet. Metal cabinets are preferred but wood is acceptable. The maximum capacity of the cabinet is 60 gallons. Metal cabinets must be made of double walled sheet iron with 1.5 inches of air space between the double walls. The internal temperature of the fire cabinet should not exceed 325°F when subjected to a 10-minute fire test.

OSHA does not specifically require signage on the fire cabinet or the door to the fire cabinet room. I would highly recommend signage as a lab best practice. See the picture below and chapter 7 for examples of fire cabinet signage. OSHA requires the presence of a portable fire extinguisher immediately outside the door to the fire cabinet room and requires all portable fire extinguishers to have an annual maintenance check to ensure they remain in good working order.

Here is a picture of my lab's fire cabinets. This is typical of most laboratory fire cabinets.

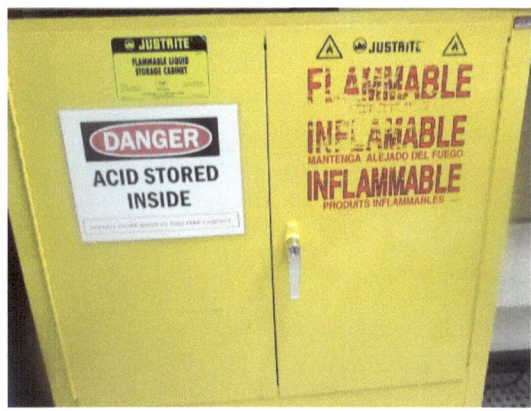

Anyone bringing chemicals out from the fire cabinet should don the appropriate PPE (gloves, lab coat, goggles, etc.) before opening the cabinet. The items being used should be transferred under a chemical hood for mixing, other preparation, etc. prior to use. If you don't have a chemical hood you could probably use a BSC cabinet for this purpose.

If your lab staff follow the chemical hazard precautions there is very little risk of a significant contamination (spills outside the chemical hood, splash in the eye, etc.). As a Laboratory BioSafety Officer, it is imperative to ensure that the lab staff are using appropriate PPE when handling toxic chemicals. Goggles will largely eliminate the risk of splashes in the eye. Impervious lab coats will largely eliminate the risk of skin contamination. However, the risk is not completely eliminated. The chemical hood should be in the same room as the fire and/or corrosive cabinets. Chemical spill kits should be present in the same room as the chemical hood, fire cabinets and corrosive cabinets. Check these spill kits for expiration dates.

OSHA requires an emergency eyewash and an emergency shower to be present in the work area if corrosive chemicals are being used. The reference is 29 CFR § 1910.151. In most labs the emergency eyewash is in the same room as the chemical hood and the emergency shower is nearby. If there is an exposure to a corrosive chemical, it is imperative to start the decontamination as soon as possible. The recommendation is that the eyewash and emergency shower should be available within 55 feet, as that is how far a person can run in 10 seconds.

The American National Standards Institute (ANSI) has made a series of recommendations in regards to emergency showers and eyewashes, but these are not regulatory requirements. One of these recommendations is annual inspection. Make sure your emergency shower and emergency eyewash have current inspection tags on them. The inspectors will be checking the flow rate, spray pattern, temperature of the water, speed of valve activation, valve remains on until shut off, etc. The emergency shower and eyewash need to pass on all the above parameters to pass inspection. Any emergency eyewash or shower that fails inspection should be repaired or replaced.

Make sure the lab staff know the location and how to operate all emergency eyewashes and showers in lab. These emergency eyewashes and showers should be turned on to let them run at least once per week to avoid buildup of stagnant water in the pipes. If you turn these on and the water that issues is brown or otherwise discolored, it means they are not being run often enough, and the frequency of checks needs to be increased. Your lab should document the emergency eyewash and shower checks.

The general procedure for use of the emergency eyewash is:

1. If a toxic chemical contaminates the eye it is imperative to start flushing as quickly as possible. The recommendation is to start within 10 seconds. If a chemical exposure to the eye occurs bring the victim to the eyewash station immediately without delay.
2. The typical eyewash station looks like a water fountain and has an activation lever. Push the activation lever. Other types of eyewash station operate with handles, etc. See the pictures on the next two pages. Once turned on the eyewash should continue to run without needing to hold pressure on the lever or handle.
3. Some types of eyewash station have a dust cover. These will typically pop off automatically once the water stream has started. If the dust covers do not pop off you will need to remove them.
4. Flush the eyes for at least 15 minutes by lowering your head into the stream of water. Hold the eyelids open using thumb and fingers. Chemical exposures in the eye are painful and this tends to cause the eyelids to spasm. The water stream will not be effective flushing the eyes if the eyelids are closed. Thus the need to hold the eyelids open with thumb and fingers. If the victim is incapacitated by intense pain others should assist the victim by bringing the victim to the eyewash and holding the victim's eyes open in the stream of water.
5. Look into the water stream to flush the eye. Roll the eyes gently up and down and from left to right to help the water reach as much of the eyeball as possible.
6. If you are wearing contact lenses, gently remove them AFTER you have started the flushing. Do not delay the flushing to remove the contact lenses.
7. Do not rub the eyes. Rubbing may embed any particulate matter in the eye. Rubbing the eyes may make the situation worse.
8. When the 15 minutes of flushing is over, turn off the eyewash station and seek medical attention immediately.

Operation of the typical eyewash station

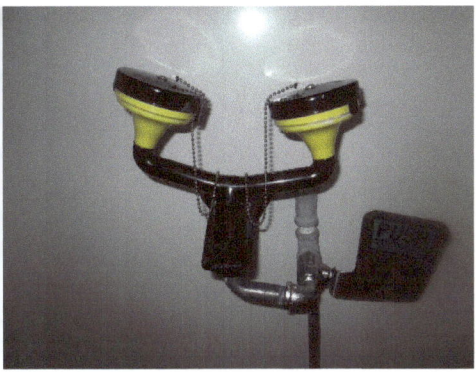

This is the appearance of the typical eyewash station with the dust covers still on.

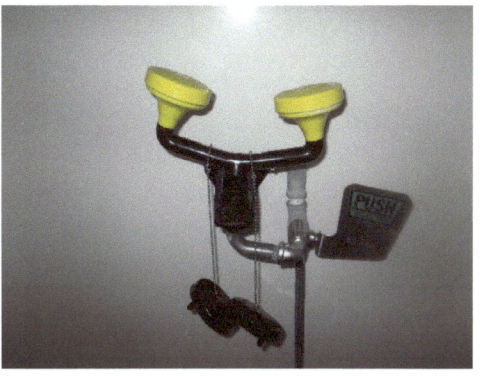

Remove the dust covers as shown here.

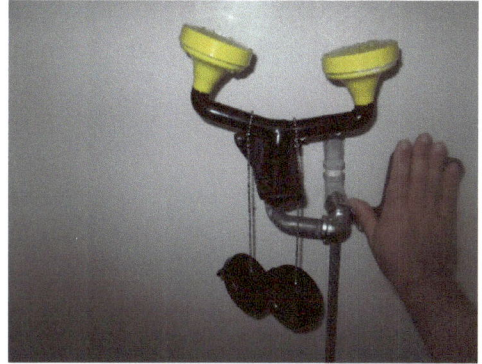

Put your hand on the activator lever.

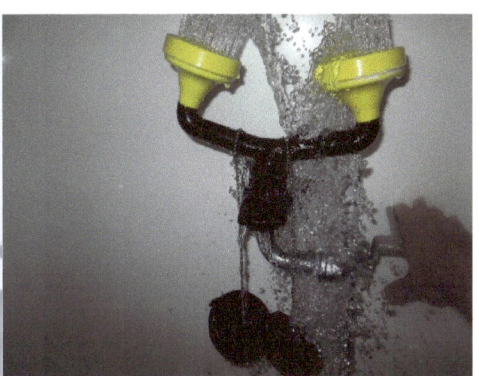

Depress the activator lever.

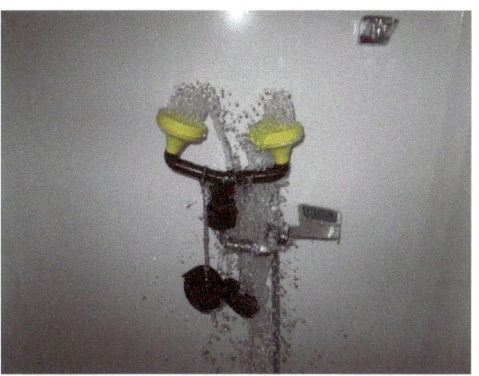

The eyewash remains on after the activator lever has been depressed.

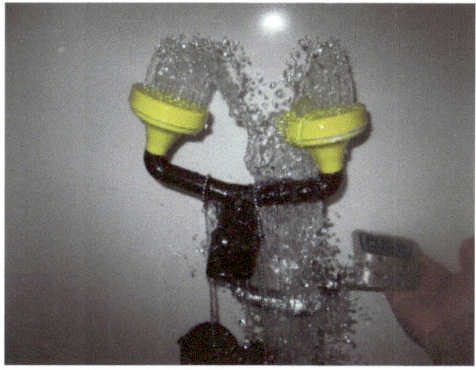

To turn off the eyewash, pull forward on the activator lever.

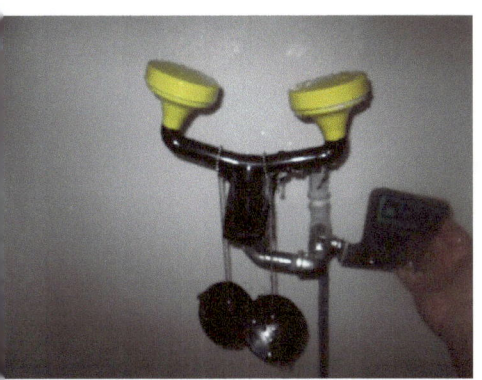

This is how the eyewash appears after being turned off.

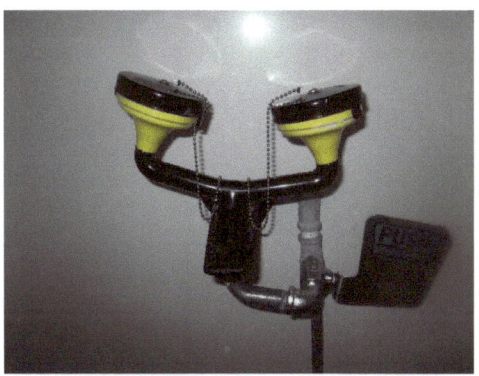

Replace the dust covers when done using the eyewash.

Drench hose used as an eyewash

The device depicted below is a drench hose. Notice the flexible hose identifying it as a drench hose. ANSI regulations state that a drench hose can be used as an emergency eyewash provided that the drench hose meets all specifications for an emergency eyewash.

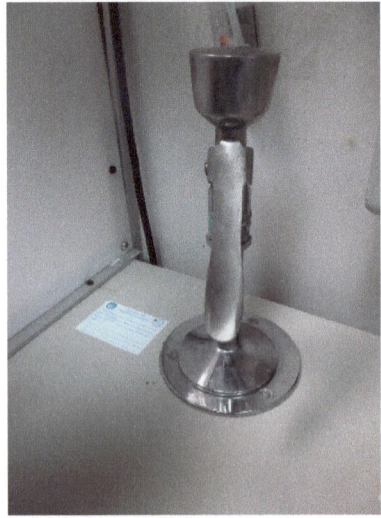

This is the appearance of a drench hose not in use.

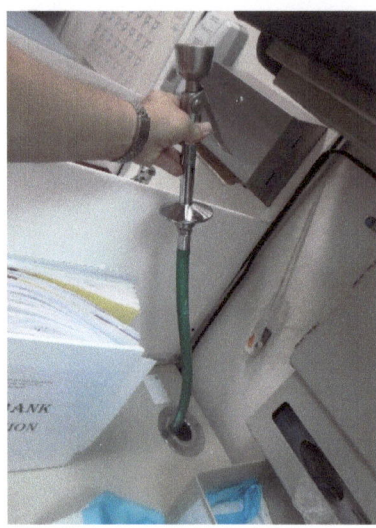

Pull up to extend the hose.

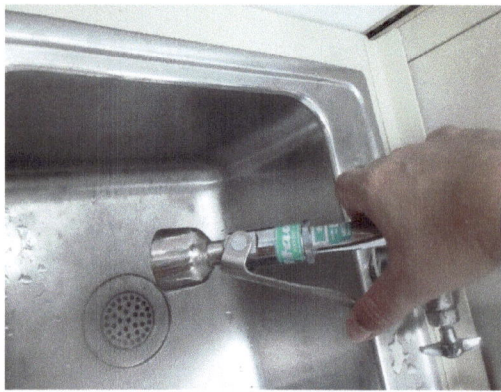

Hold the lever.

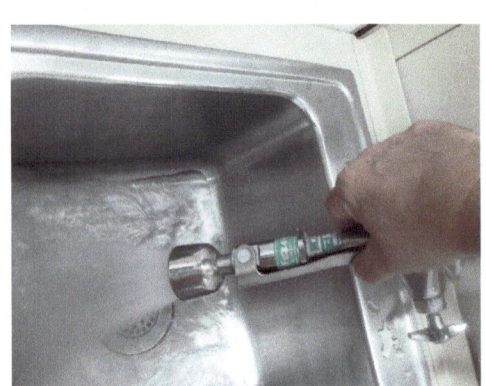

Depress the lever.

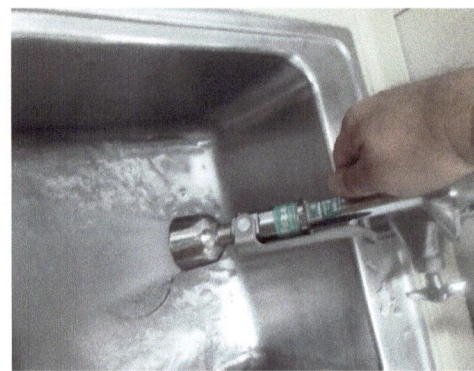

Once depressed the lever remains in and the water continues to run until turned off.

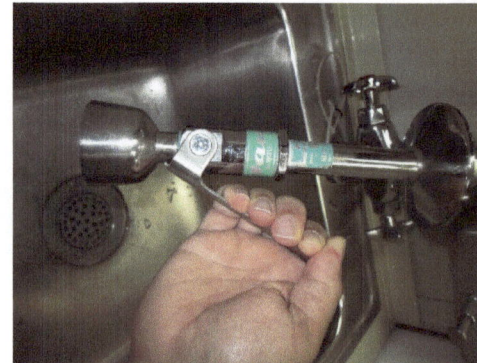

Turn the drench hose off by pulling the lever out.

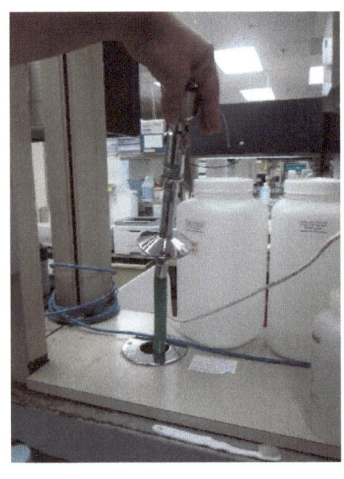

When done move the drench hose back into the vertical position and push down to retract the hose.

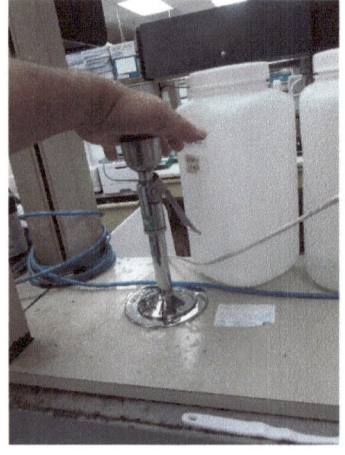

Be careful not to touch the lever when replacing the drench hose or you may spill water on the counter as shown in this photo.

Operation of the typical emergency shower

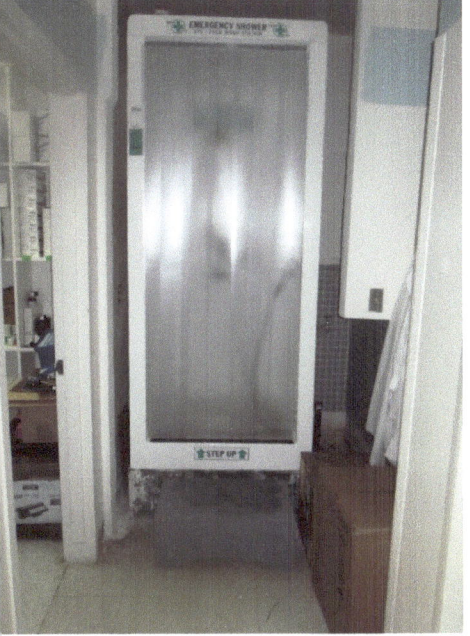

This is the typical emergency shower stall.

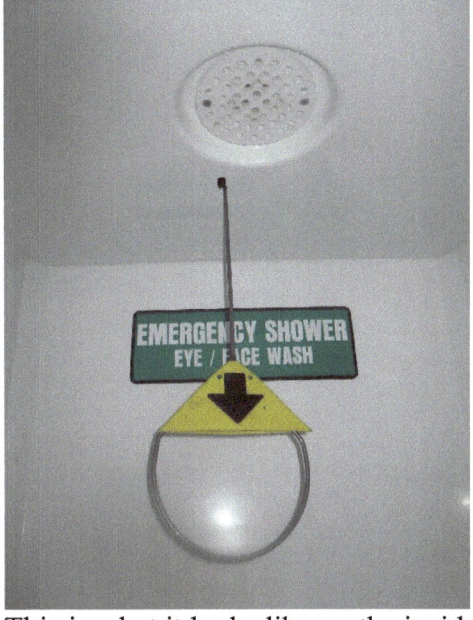

This is what it looks like on the inside.

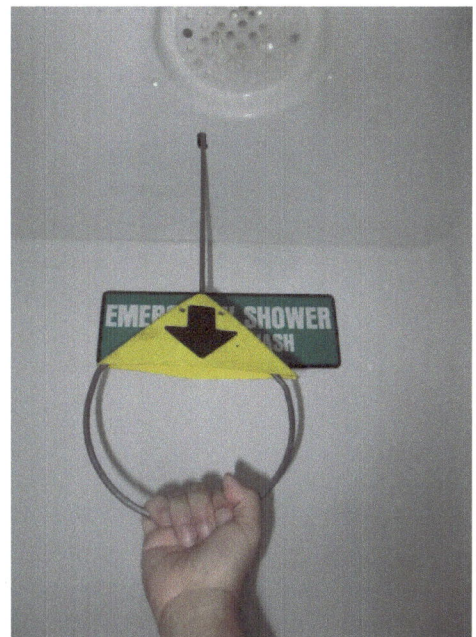

Pull the handle to turn it on.

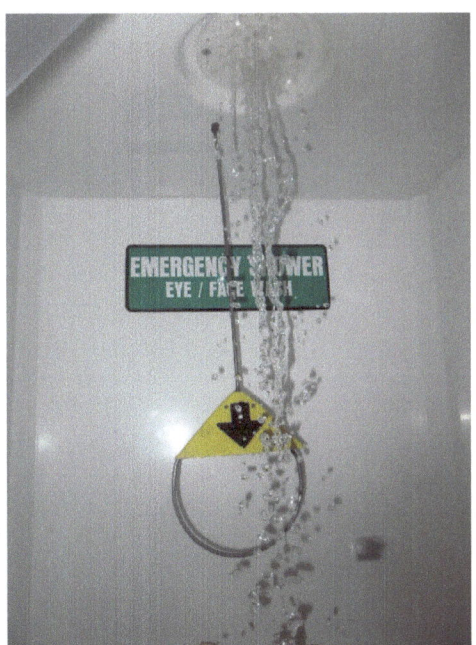

Once the handle is pulled the shower runs continuously.

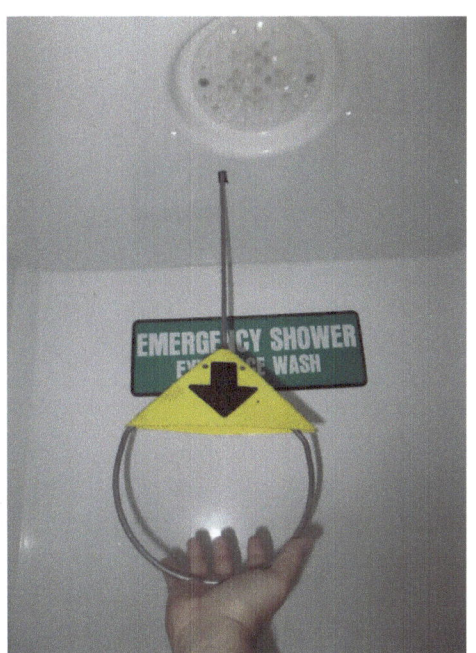

To turn off the emergency shower, push up on the handle.

The general procedure for the use of the emergency shower is:

1. If a toxic chemical contaminates the skin it is important to wash it off as quickly as possible. The longer a chemical remains on the skin the more time it has to do damage. If a chemical exposure to the skin occurs bring the victim to the emergency shower as soon as possible. Do not delay.

2. The typical emergency shower station looks like a small household shower stall. It typically has a pull lever. Other types of emergency shower look like a freestanding shower-head in lab without the associated stall. When turned on this freestanding shower head will flood the lab with water. Do not hesitate to use this type of emergency shower. The flood in lab can be mopped up later. Once turned on the shower should continue to run without having to continuously pull the lever. See the pictures on the previous page.
3. Remove any contaminated clothing and/or PPE while under the shower. An assistant may need to hold up a blanket or sheet for privacy for the person undressing under the emergency shower, Wear gloves and other PPE when handling the victim's contaminated clothes. Place contaminated clothes in plastic bags for chemical hazard disposal.
4. Flush the affected skin area for at least 15 minutes. Make sure the eyes are above the level of the flush area so that contaminated flush water does NOT enter the eyes.
5. When the 15 minutes of flushing is over, turn off the emergency shower by pushing up on the pull lever. Seek medical attention immediately.

OSHA requires exposure monitoring for some chemicals. In the typical clinical laboratory, formalin is the only chemical that requires personnel exposure monitoring. OSHA gives the formaldehyde monitoring regulatory requirements at 29 CFR § 1910.1048. To briefly summarize: The employer must identify all employees who may be exposed to formaldehyde. The employer is required to perform initial monitoring and periodic monitoring for formaldehyde exposure. The employer may monitor the exposure of all employees potentially exposed to formaldehyde or a representative sampling. The monitoring must be repeated every 6 months if the results are at or above the action level. The action level is 0.5 Parts Per Million (PPM) formaldehyde on a Time Weighted Average (TWA) concentration for 8 hours. The monitoring must be repeated every year if the results are above the Short Term Exposure Limit (STEL) of 2 PPM formaldehyde for 15 minutes. If results are below the action level and STEL for 2 consecutive measurements at least 7 days apart the monitoring can be dropped. The employer must notify each employee of his or her results within 15 days of receipt of the results.

This regulatory requirement is typically met by contracting out to a company that deals with formalin monitoring badges. The company sends the badges, the employees wear them for a set amount of time, typically 15 minutes or 8 hours, then the badges are returned to the company for processing and evaluation. The company will send you the formalin monitoring reports typically a few weeks after receiving the badges back. If the permissible exposure limit (PEL) is not exceeded, all you have to do is sign the report and file it.

If the PEL is exceeded, you have to mitigate the formalin exposure. Typical mitigations for formalin exposure include requiring all pouring of formalin under a hood, checking and increasing the air flow on the hood, venting the hood exhaust away from lab, ensuring the formalin is mixed properly (10% concentration is not exceeded), increasing the ventilation in the histology room, etc.

If you can't mitigate the formalin exposure you will need to make everyone working in histology wear respirator masks while at work. I have never seen a histology department where everyone wears respirator masks, so I assume that all histology departments nationwide have adequate formalin exposure mitigation in place.

Chemical fume hoods share many similarities to biosafety cabinets (BSC). Both chemical fume hoods and BSC are enclosed, ventilated devices designed to protect the user from hazards. As discussed in the next chapter, it is possible to use some types of BSC as fume hoods (i.e. work with hazardous chemicals in a biosafety cabinet). However, the typical chemical fume hood can't be used for working with infectious organisms for reasons that will be discussed in the next chapter.

Here is a picture of the typical chemical fume hood and a diagram showing the airflow:

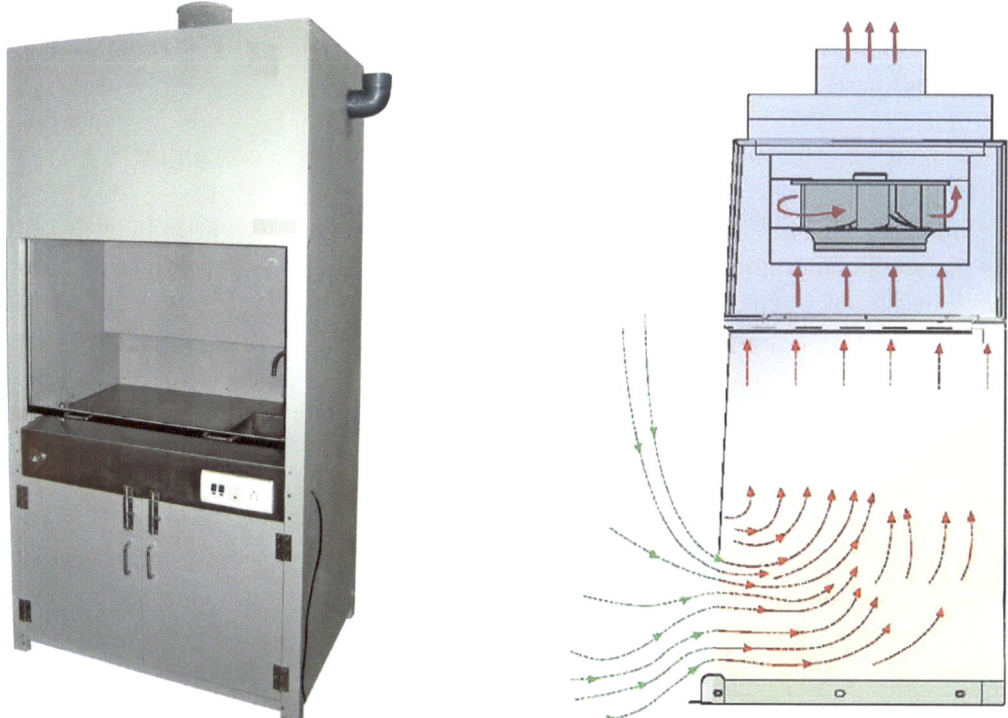

Chemical fume hoods and biosafety cabinets share the same basic design. They enclose five sides of the work surface. Only the front is open, and the front opening is typically partially covered by a movable window called a sash. The user's arms are inserted through the front opening. The airflow in the hood prevents any contaminated air from reaching the user, protecting the user from the hazards within the hood.

There are significant differences between chemical fume hoods and BSC. The typical laboratory chemical fume hood exhausts 100% of air outside the building. Removing volatile chemicals from the air is difficult (this would require a "scrubber") and generally not worthwhile. It is much easier to exhaust the chemically contaminated air outside of the building. In contrast the typical BSC recirculates air after filtering the air through HEPA filters to purify it. Before and after working in a BSC you must disinfect it thoroughly. However, the cleanup before and after use of a chemical fume hood tends not to be as meticulous.

There are many similarities between chemical fume hoods and biosafety cabinets. They should all be located in areas of low air flow (away from windows, doors, walkways, etc.) as airflow from outside sources can disrupt the airflow in the cabinet/hood. They should all be certified annually by a qualified inspector. They should all have alarms for low air flow. I will go into much more detail on this in the next chapter. The best practices given in the next chapter for use of BSC also largely apply to the use of chemical fume hoods.

Chapter 6 – Laboratory Biosafety containment levels and biosafety cabinets

Laboratory Biosafety containment refers exclusively to biologic hazards (infectious organisms and specimens). This is not used for chemical or other hazards.

There are four levels of biosafety, BSL-1 to BSL-4 in increasing order of containment.

BSL-1 is used with organisms that are nonpathogenic (i.e. do not cause disease in healthy humans). In this setting only minimal containment is needed. The lab workers should wear gloves and lab coats, but the work can be done on open benches without needing biosafety cabinets. This is used exclusively for environmental and veterinary testing. Clinical laboratories must use BSL-2 or higher.

BSL-2 is the typical biosafety level of the small hospital or public health lab. This level is used for moderately pathogenic organisms. In addition to the requirements of BSL-1 above, lab staff must have specific training on handling specimens. Access to lab is controlled. All sharp items must be handled with great care to avoid needlesticks. The lab may require vaccinations of workers. A biosafety manual is mandatory. Waste is decontaminated before disposal. All work capable of producing aerosols must be done in a biosafety cabinet.

BSL-3 is used for serious pathogens that can spread by the respiratory route. In addition to the BSL-2 requirements above, solid front PPE (a wraparound gown or coveralls) is required before entering the room with the BSC. There must be negative pressure with air only allowed to flow from the clean areas of lab into the room with the BSC. Exhaust air from the BSC room must be decontaminated and not allowed to enter lab. The requirements for doffing and disposing the gown on exit are more stringent than for BSL-2. Thus, BSL-3 typically entails an anteroom for donning and doffing PPE adjacent to the room with the BSL cabinet.

BSL-4 is used for extremely dangerous pathogens. In addition to the BSL-3 requirements above, there should be a Class III Biosafety cabinet or else a full body suit with positive air pressure. Usually a BSL-4 lab will be in its own isolated building with surrounding security perimeter. The lab staff are required to completely change clothes on entry and shower on exit. All materials are decontaminated prior to exit from the facility.

The terms BSL-2+ and Enhanced BSL-2 refer to the use of BSL-2 equipment with BSL-3 practices. This is not really an official or recognized level of containment. It is typically used at older facilities that were built as a BSL-2 but want to expand their testing to organisms or test systems that require more containment.

For example, one Public Health lab I have visited was built as a BSL-2 but wanted to add DNA testing on an ABI-7500 analyzer. They did this by putting in BSL-3 practices. When processing the specimen the lab tech will work under a BSL-2 hood. Another lab tech will be wearing clean PPE and waiting behind the lab tech doing the work. When done manipulating the specimen, the lab tech working at the hood will decontaminate the exterior of the specimen container and hand it off to the clean lab tech standing in the same room. The practices are BSL-3 but the equipment is BSL-2.

This is not the optimal way of doing things, it would have been best if this lab was built as a BSL-3 from the start. However, this does meet regulations and allows the lab to perform an expanded range of testing. If you are planning to set up a BSL-2 or BSL-2+ lab be careful that the organisms you will be testing are not really BSL-3 or higher. For example, culturing of tuberculosis requires BSL-3 or higher. You cannot attempt this with BSL-2+. Know the BSL level requirement of all organisms your lab tests.

For BSL-2 and higher, the front door to the room containing the BSL cabinet should be kept locked by a self-closing door. Swipe card locks are preferred over key locks, as swipe card locks record information on whose swipe card was used to enter and when. BSL-3 and higher typically have a security camera monitoring the activities in the BSL room. Signage is required on the front of the BSL room, such as the following:

BSL2

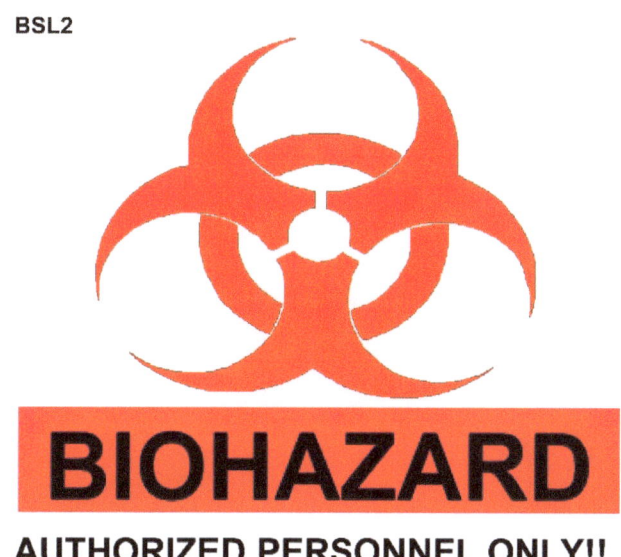

As mentioned above, BSL-2 and higher requires that all work capable of aerosolizing samples must be done in a biosafety cabinet (BSC). This includes centrifugation, aliquoting, sonicating, etc. of a specimen or culture. BSC come in three classes. The three classes of BSC differ in their flow rates, direction of air flow, and location of the High Efficiency Particulate Air (HEPA) filters used to decontaminate the exhaust air. Here is a picture of a Class I BSC and a diagram of the airflow:

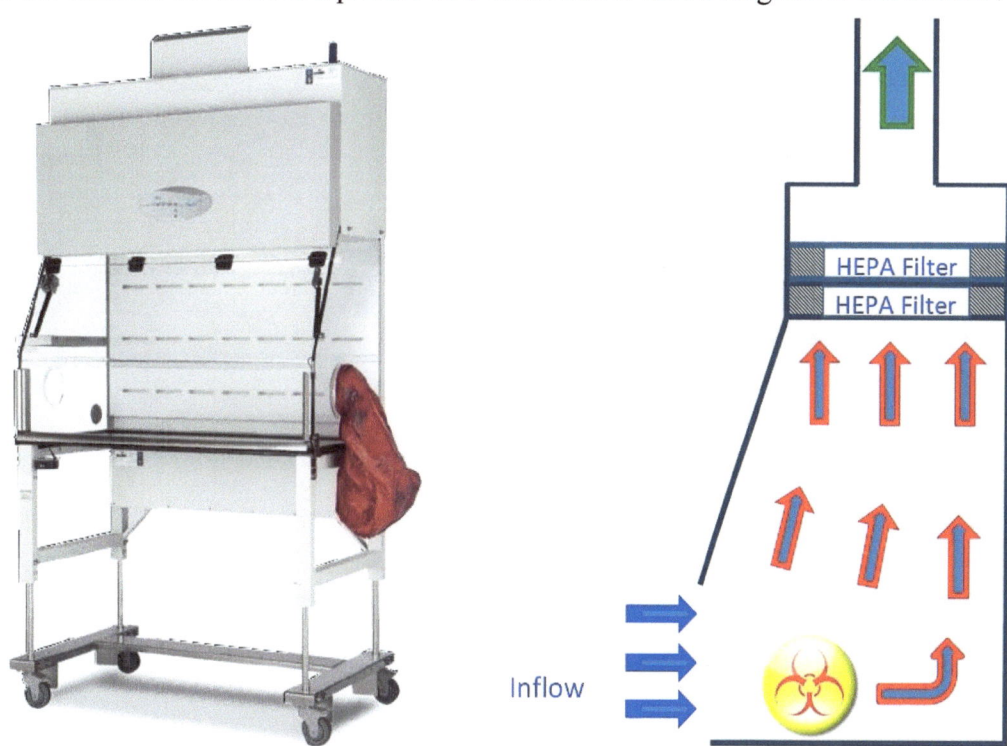

Class I BSC's are most often associated with BSL-1. This type of hood maintains an inward flow of air of at least 75 feet per minute (22.6 meters per minute). However the direction of airflow is entirely inward. This protects the operator from contamination by the pathogen, but does NOT protect the sample being manipulated from contamination by the inward flow of air. Hence, this type of BSC is not typically used for BSL-2 and higher.

Class II BSC's have an inward flow of air and another downward stream of HEPA filtered air to protect the sample from contamination by the air being drawn into the BSC. This type of BSC is most commonly associated with BSL-2 and BSL-3. Class II is broken down into five types: A1, A2, B1, B2 and C1.

Here is a picture of a class II BSC and an airflow diagram of a Class II type A BSC:

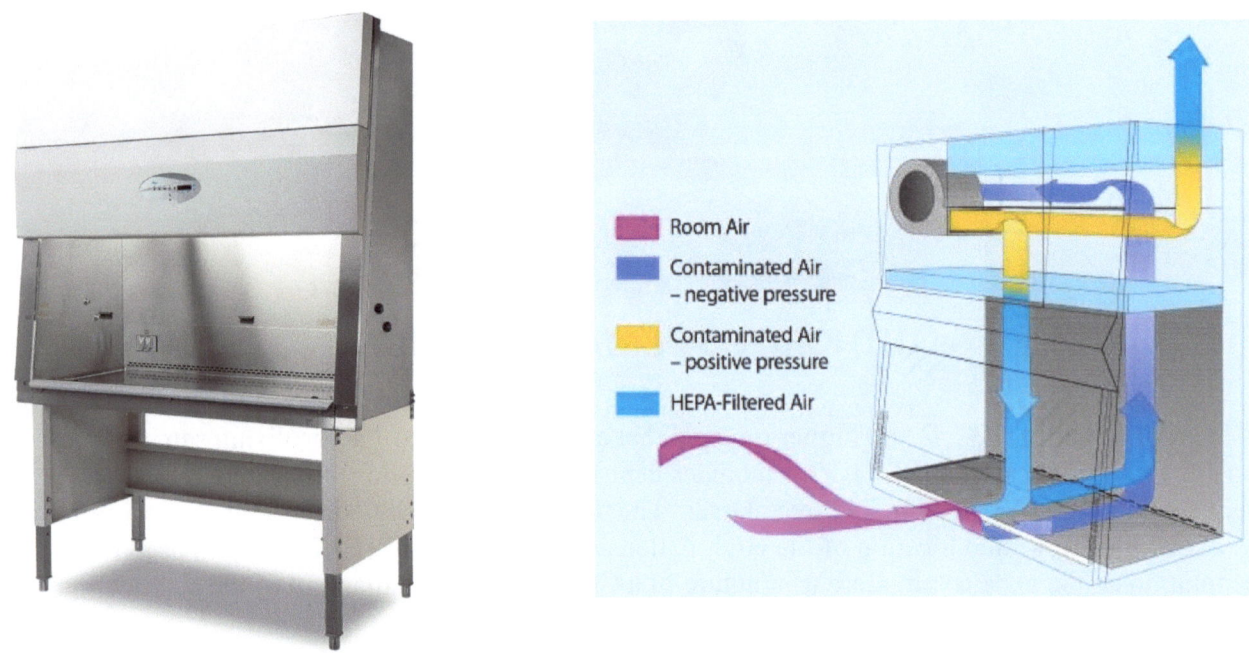

Class II type A1 BSC's have a minimum inward airflow of at least 75 feet per minute (22.6 meters per minute). About 70% of the inflow air is recirculated inside the BSC.

Class II type A2 BSC's have a minimum inward airflow of at least 100 feet per minute (30.5 meters per minute) but are otherwise similar to type A1. Class II type A2 BSC's are the most common biosafety cabinets in use in clinical microbiology laboratories and represent the vast majority of BSC's I have ever seen. Because Class II type A1 and type A2 BSC's recirculate air they are not optimal for use as a chemical fume hood. If used with volatile chemicals, the vapors could build up in the recirculated air increasing the risk of fire or explosion.

Here is an airflow diagram of a Class II type B BSC. This type of BSC will look the same from the exterior as the BSC pictured on the previous page:

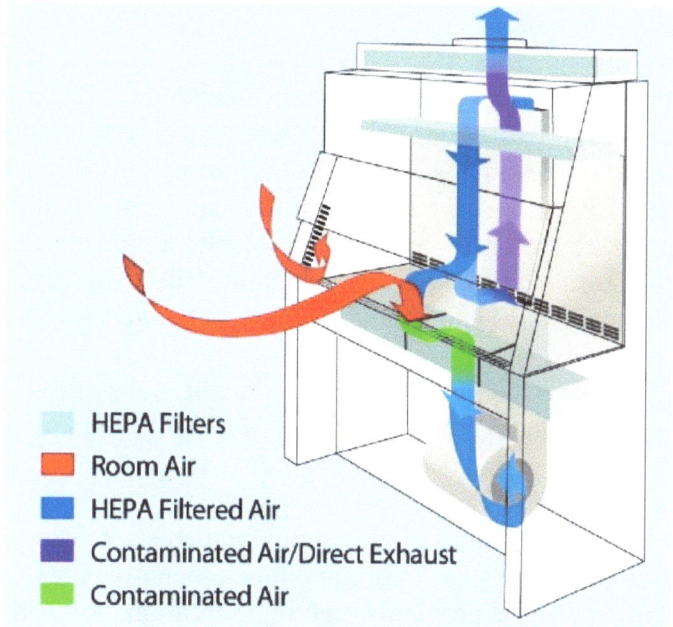

Class II type B1 and B2 BSC's have a minimum inward airflow of at least 100 feet per minute (30.5 meters per minute). They have less recirculation of air. Type B1 recirculates 60% or less of the inflow air and Type B2 does not recirculate any inflow air. These BSC can also be used as chemical fume hoods, since they do not have the problem of vapor buildup seen with Class II type A1 and A2 BSC's.

Class II type C1 is essentially the same as a type B except that it has been modified so that it can run its internal fans to purify air indefinitely in case of hospital-wide power or ventilating system failure.

Here is a diagram of a Class III BSC. There is no airflow in this type of BSC:

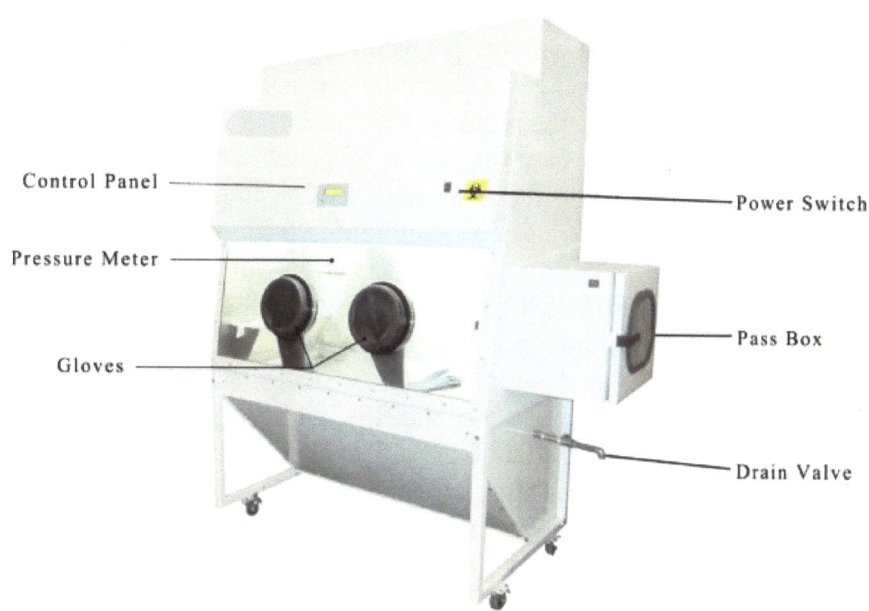

Class III BSC's have an airtight enclosure. The specimens are manipulated through gloves attached to the front of the enclosure. This is typically only needed for BSL-4 containment.

All BSC's have HEPA filters and a gauge on the BSC measuring the pressure drop across the filter. Any cabinet lacking these features should not be used as a BSC. The pressure drop across the HEPA filters differs from one BSC to another.

The BSC should come from the manufacturer with a recommended range for the pressure drop reading on this gauge. The lab tech operating the BSC should always check this reading and document it before beginning work in the BSC. If the reading is higher than the acceptable range (pressure drop too large) it indicates blockage of the HEPA filters, typically by particulate matter that has built up over time as the filter operates. If the pressure drop is lower than the acceptable range (pressure drop too small) it indicates the HEPA filter has torn a hole or otherwise lost integrity. Any BSC with this pressure drop reading out of range should not be used and should be taken out of service until it can be repaired.

Repair work on BSC's is typically done by an outside contractor, not by lab. This includes changing HEPA filters, replacing fan motors, etc. The BSC will need to be decontaminated prior to this work. Typically the contractor will perform this decontamination as well.

The BSC should be certified before use and at least annually thereafter. The certifier will typical check for HEPA filter leaks, intake air velocity, exhaust air velocity, negative pressure, ventilation rate, airflow smoke patterns, alarms, electric problems, lighting, vibration, noise, etc. The certifier will typically place a tag on the BSC stating the date of certification and the expiration date. Any BSC that fails on any of the above parameters should be taken out of service until it can be repaired.

All Class I and Class II BSC's depend on inward air flow to protect the user from contamination. Anything that disrupts the inward flow of air should be strictly prohibited in the BSC room. This includes:

1. Placing anything over the front or rear grille. A large object placed on the front or rear grille will block the BSC's intake or exhaust of air, respectively. This should set off an alarm. Blocking the front grille is a worst case scenario for this type of BSC, since it allows contaminated air to blow directly into the face of the person seated at the BSC. Blocking the rear grille is not quite as bad, but should still be avoided.
2. Some BSC's have a movable window pane called a window sash. In these BSC opening the window sash too wide or closing it will disrupt the airflow in the BSC and set off the BSC's alarms. If this happens, move the window sash back to a middling position. Do not close this sash while the BSC's fans are running as this could cause the fan motors to burn out.
3. Anyone walking by the BSC will cause currents of air that could disrupt the BSC's airflow. It is for this reason that BSC's should have their own room separate from the rest of the lab and should never be put in lab's common areas with heavy traffic of people walking through. Keep the door to the BSC room locked while the BSC is in use.
4. The operator moving his or her arms in and out of the BSC frequently. Before starting work in the BSC, you should load all supplies, culture plates, etc. into the BSC. You don't want to keep moving your arms in and out of the BSC while working with live cultures. If you must move your arms out of the BSC, use a directly in and out motion. Do mot move your arms sideways as this generates more air currents.
5. Electric fans should not be allowed in the BSC room.
6. Most BSC rooms do not have a window. If your BSC room has a window, make sure it is locked in the closed position before starting work in the BSC.
7. Lab equipment that creates air movement (vacuum filters, etc.) should not be kept in the BSC room.

8. The incoming air from air supply ducts can disrupt the BSC's air flow. The BSC room needs to be highly ventilated, the OSHA recommendation is 4 to 12 Air Changes per Hour (ACH), but the incoming air should not be aimed at the BSC. The BSC should be situated in a corner of the BSC room away from air supply ducts.
9. Open flames. These are not permitted in the BSC.

Safe operation of a BSC requires prior education, training and competency testing. The typical procedure for use of the BSC is to wash your hands and don proper PPE prior to entering the BSC room, lock the BSC room door immediately after entry, close and lock any windows, make sure the BSC's movable sash (if any) is in the proper position, check any drain valves, turn on the BSC's fans, wait at least 10 minutes to allow for air filtration in the BSC, check the gauge reading to make sure it is acceptable, check the alarm and document this information in the logbook as required (date, time, guage reading, results of alarm test, etc.). Disinfect the interior surfaces of the BSC and load all necessary supplies, reagents, cultures, etc. into the BSC. Do not load anything into the BSC that you will not be using. Before starting work, double-check that you have loaded everything into the BSC you will need during your work. You don't want to open live cultures and then realize you have left the pipette tips in the next room over.

Keep the clean and the contaminated items as separate work areas at least 12 inches apart from each other inside the BSC. Do not mix clean and contaminated items together as a single work area. Do not place anything within 4 inches of the front or rear grille. Equipment that can generate aerosols (centrifuges, etc.) should be kept at the back of the BSC. Adjust the chair so that you are at a comfortable level relative to the work you will be doing and your head is above the level of the BSC's front opening. Start your work with the clean items and then move to the contaminated work when done with the clean work.

When done with your work remove all unnecessary items from the BSC and discard all waste. Any waste that has been inside a BSC is assumed to be contaminated and must go in red bag trash or sharps containers. Never put any waste from the BSC in the white bag trash. Disinfect the interior surfaces of the BSC. Any equipment or supplies put in the BSC must be disinfected on removal from the BSC by swabbing the surfaces with bleach or alcohol.

Let the BSC's fans run for at least 10 minutes after you have completed your work. This will allow time for the BSC to filter out any remaining organisms from the air in the BSC. When done, turn off the BSC's fans, properly dispose of your PPE in the red bag trash and wash your hands.

Some older models of BSC's come with ultraviolet (UV) lights for sterilization. This practice is highly discouraged for two reasons. First, the UV light has been associated with eye damage and cataracts in lab staff. Second, the UV light bulb tends to accumulate dust and dirt over time rendering it ineffective for sterilization. Even if your BSC has a UV light you should not use it and instead use bleach or alcohol for disinfection when done working in the BSC.

Avoid clutter in the BSC. Do not leave unnecessary items stored in the BSC when not in use. Do not store items on top of the BSC.

Most hospital and public health laboratories store small amounts of flammable and/or hazardous chemicals. Regulations require these to be stored in fire and/or corrosive cabinets when not in use. All fire and corrosive cabinets should be marked with appropriate signage. This includes the NFPA sign discussed in a prior chapter. This does not include the globally harmonized pictograms, as these are typically only used for shipping, not storage in a cabinet. Examples of the appropriate signage to use, in addition to the NFPA sign are:

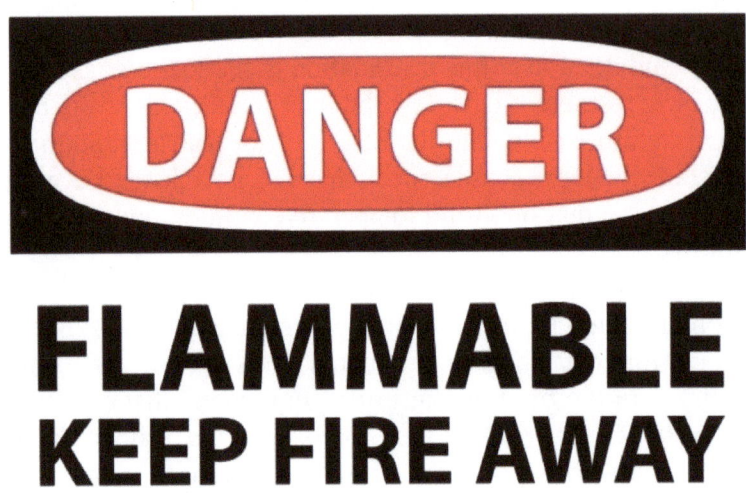

Only hazardous and/or flammable chemicals belong in these cabinets. There is no point in keeping lab's sodium bicarbonate in the fire cabinet, since it is neither flammable nor toxic.

Some types of hazardous chemicals should not be stored in the same cabinet, for example acids and bases. If the acids and bases ever mix, they could react violently. Thus acids and bases should be stored in separate cabinets.

Do not store oxidizers (e.g. iodine, ferric chloride) in the same cabinet with flammables. If they mix they could ignite. Do not store acids in the same cabinet with chemicals that could react with acid producing toxic gasses (e.g. sodium cyanide).

TEST – Let's say you are doing a risk assessment. You open up this fire cabinet or any other fire cabinet with similar signage on the front:

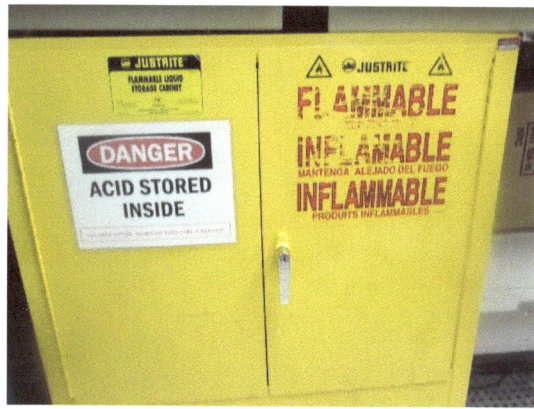

and you find the following. What is wrong with this picture?

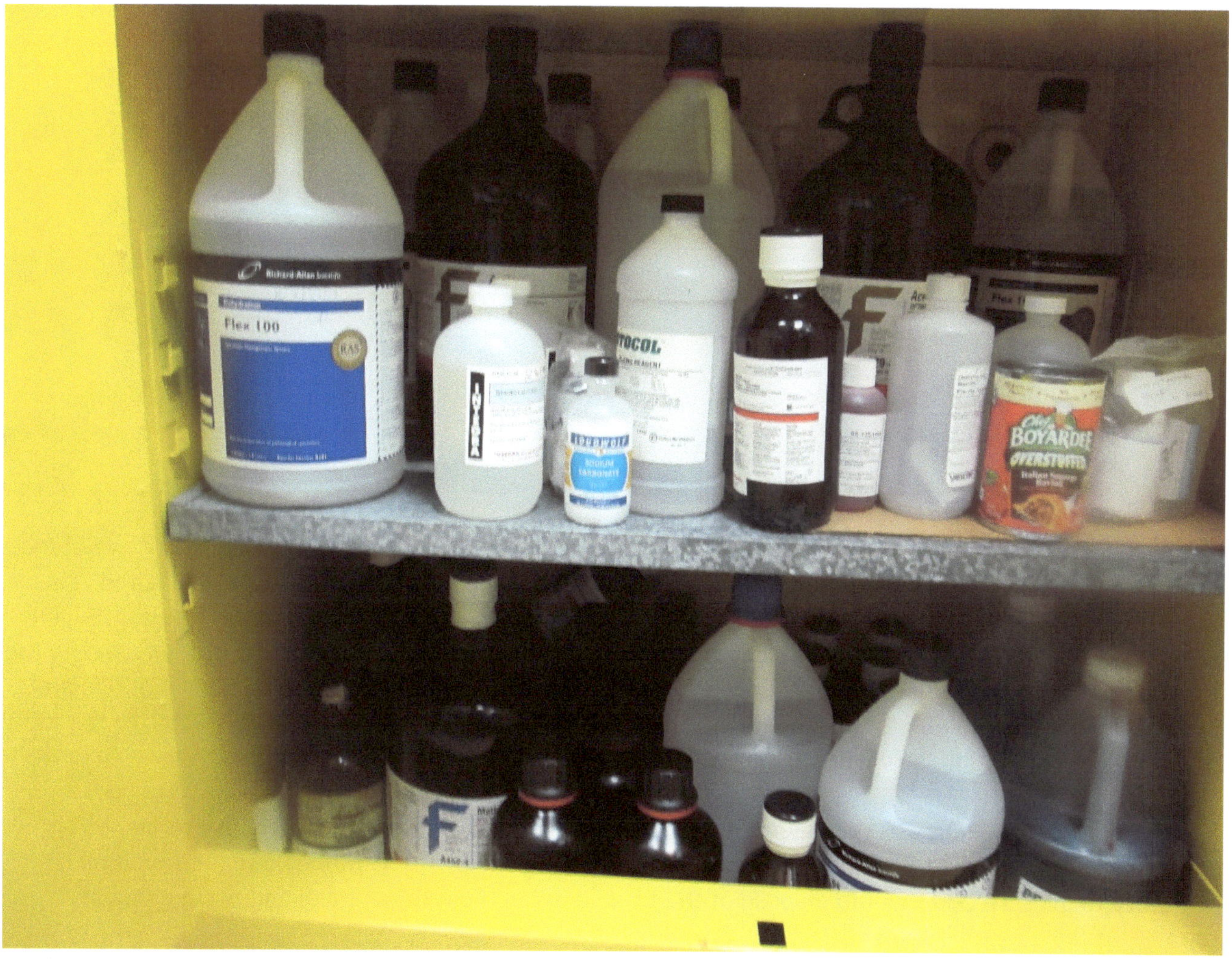

HINT: This is a staged photo. I opened up the fire cabinet in my own lab, put two items inside that do not belong, took this photo, then immediately removed the two items that do not belong and closed up the fire cabinet. Can you find the two items that do not belong?

ANSWER:

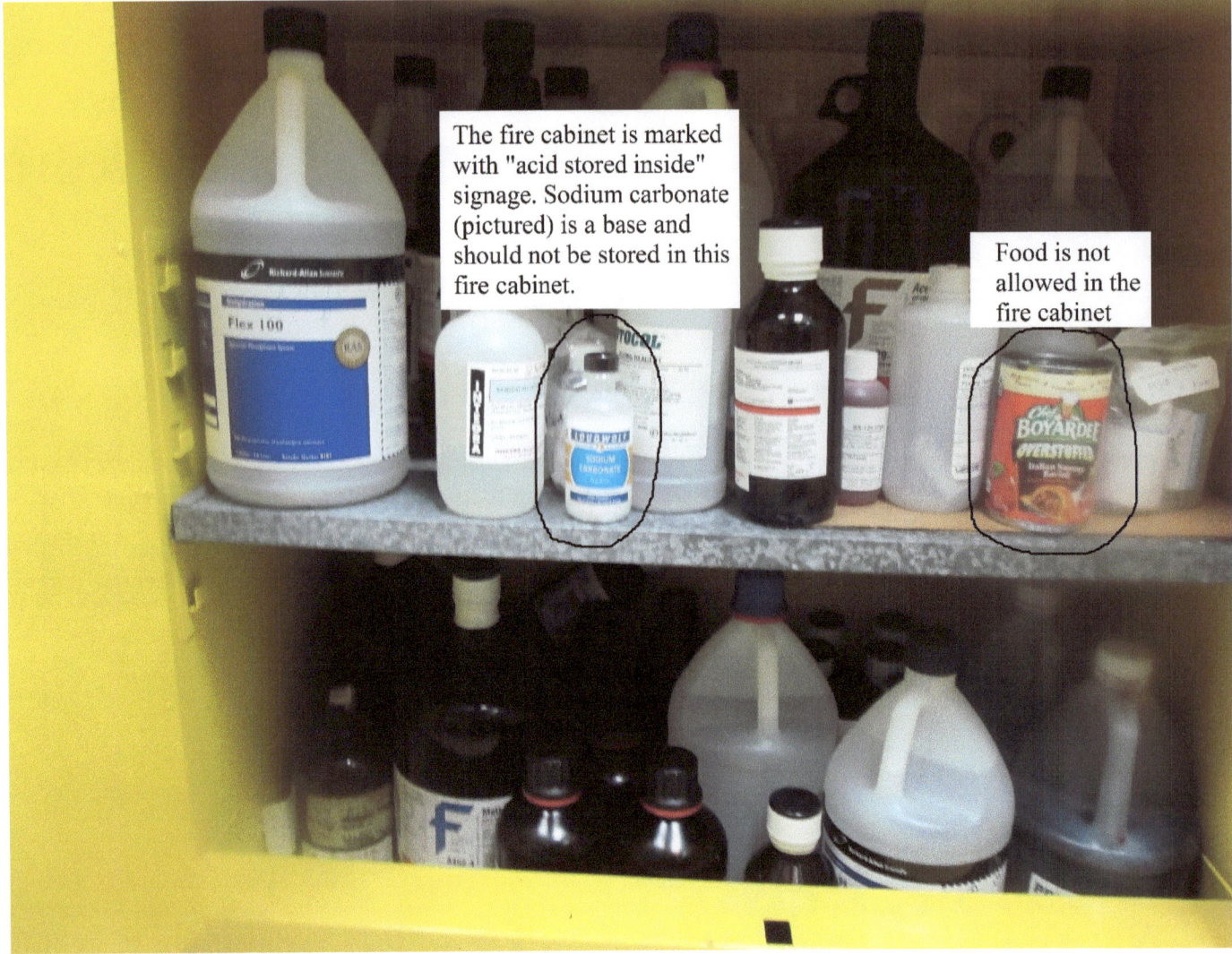

The fire cabinet is marked with "acid stored inside" signage. Sodium carbonate (pictured) is a base and should not be stored in this fire cabinet.

Food is not allowed in the fire cabinet

Food should only be allowed in lab's break room and not allowed in lab's work areas. In my experience it is not uncommon to find food items stored in places where they are not supposed to be stored. This is typically a problem in the phlebotomy refrigerator used to store glucola for the glucose testing. I have seen a few instances where empty fire cabinets not in use for chemical storage were instead used by the lab staff for storing personal items including bags of potato chips. The scenarios described above are not a risk of contamination to the lab staff and I will politely tell the lab staff to please remove the food and do not store food in lab's work areas.

I have not seen food items in specimen refrigerators or fire cabinets that contained hazardous chemicals. If this were to ever happen, it would be a risk of chemical or biological contamination. If this were to ever happen I would dispose of the food items in the red bag trash and write incident reports for the lab staff involved.

The sodium carbonate pictured above is typical of an accidental storage of incompatible items in a fire cabinet. You should open up your fire cabinets at least every 6 months and check inside to make sure no one has put incompatible chemicals together in the same fire cabinet.

Chapter 8 – Physical hazards in lab

The broadest definition of a physical hazard is anything in the environment that can cause harm. In a clinical laboratory this includes electric wiring, slippery floors, injuries from lab equipment, burns from the autoclave, carpal tunnel syndrome from your keyboard, and a long list of other potential hazards.

Falls are the most common cause of occupational injury. Labs should not have rugs or carpets. The main problem with rugs and carpets in lab is that they can harbor microorganisms. They are also a risk for slips and falls. On a smooth tile floor, your risk of falls increases considerable when the floor is wet. Make sure housekeeping does all their mopping and other cleaning at night when few people are present in lab. The only mopping during the day should occur if there is a spill. If there is any liquid on the floor, have it mopped up immediately and/or set down "Wet Floor" warning signs. Keep all walkways clear of obstructions.

Machine injuries are probably the second most common cause of occupational injury. This is less common in lab as compared to other occupations. For example, with most centrifuges the lid cannot be opened until the centrifuge stops. Make sure the lab staff do not attempt to defeat the safety mechanisms. For all equipment with an emergency shut off, the lab staff operating the equipment should be familiar with how to operate the emergency shut off.

In my experience, the most common occupational problem in lab is carpal tunnel syndrome. I have worked at labs where 5% to 10% of the lab staff have carpal tunnel syndrome. Make sure lab gets ergonomic keyboards for all lab staff. The lab staff with carpal tunnel syndrome may need additional accommodations including a more ergonomic desk and/or chair, longer breaks at work, reassignment to areas where they don't have to do as much typing, etc.

Some laboratories have compressed gas cylinders, typically carbon dioxide for bacterial incubation. Hospital regulations require all compressed gas cylinders to be chained down so they don't go flying if the valve is accidentally broken off. The following are best practices involving compressed gas cylinders: All compressed gas cylinders should be secured in an upright position away from sparks, open flame, electricity, etc. Empty cylinders should be stored separately from full cylinders.

In the typical hospital lab, the lab staff do not change the compressed gas cylinders when empty; instead the hospital's maintenance department is called in to replace an empty tank with a full one, check the pressure on the newly installed tank, check the valve and regulator for leaks, secure the valve cap on the empty tank, remove the empty tank from lab, etc. In my experience, the lab staff do not touch or manipulate the compressed gas cylinders in lab. They will call the hospital's maintenance department immediately if a problem develops with a compressed gas cylinder.

In my experience thermal injuries are rare in lab. Burns from the autoclave are uncommon and frostbite from the -70°C freezer is almost unheard of. Make sure the lab has thermal PPE (thermal gloves) and the lab staff are aware of the requirement to use thermal PPE for removing any items from the autoclave and freezers below -20°C.

At one time in the remote past most Biosafety Cabinets (BSC) had built-in ultraviolet (UV) lights to perform sterilization. There were reports of this causing eye damage and cataracts to lab staff. Most modern day BSC do not have UV lights. If you have an older model of BSC that still has a UV light, I would recommend NOT using the UV light for sterilization and instead disinfect the BSC surfaces with bleach or alcohol.

All electric equipment in lab should have a tag applied annually by the hospital's maintenance department. Check all these tags to make sure they are current and not expired. When the hospital's maintenance department inspects these items and applies tags they will be checking that the equipment is properly grounded, no frayed electric cords, etc.

Check all lab equipment for exposed electric wiring. Any lab equipment with any type of electric problem should be taken out of service (unplugged) until the problem can be fixed. Do not use flexible extension cords in lab. Flexible extension cords are both an electric hazard and a trip/fall hazard.

Other occupational hazards including noise, confined spaces, lasers, asphyxiation, vibrating machinery, etc. are not usually a problem in clinical laboratories. The situations and equipment that produce these types of problems are more typical of heavy industry and not typical of clinical labs.

Chapter 9 – Lab security including biosecurity, door locks and swipe cards

Lab security is primarily designed to prevent the unauthorized access to lab's chemicals, biological specimens and patient records. Other considerations including prevention of theft, sabotage, vandalism, etc. are part of lab security, but are generally considered to be lower priority. Lab biosecurity is a subset of lab security and represents measures to prevent unauthorized access to infectious materials.

Security measures can be either physical (for example swipe card locks on doors), electronic (for example password protecting all data) or operational (for example vetting of prospective employees). The lab security plan should include physical security (i.e. controlling access to the laboratory). The most obvious route of entry is the front door to lab. This should have a swipe card lock. Also consider security cameras for lab's front door. The video monitoring system should provide permanent storage of the video so it can be retrieved later if there is ever a need to document who accessed the front door.

In higher security labs (i.e. BSL-3 and higher) there is likely to be a guard checking ID's in person at lab's front door. There may also be a security call "Panic button" at the lab's front door that if activated sounds an alarm and brings the entire hospital's security forces running to lab.

Most labs have emergency exits at the back. Check these to make sure the alarm sounds when opened, these doors are automatically closing and self-locking, etc. If your lab is on the ground floor, window access is also a concern. Before you put bars on the windows, ensure that there will be adequate emergency egress (fire exits).

As Lab BSO you will enforce the physical security rules on the lab – No unauthorized visitors. Do not allow anyone into lab without a swipe card or visitor's pass. Do not lend your swipe card and/or keys to anyone. Report anyone asking to borrow your swipe card and/or keys. Anyone who does not have a swipe card or visitor's pass will need to sign in at the Security Office and receive a visitor's pass before entering lab. Make sure your hospital's Security Office has a policy stating who is allowed to visit lab and who is not. Anyone at increased risk (immunosuppressed, pregnant, etc.) should be restricted from lab.

Electronic security involves password security (no sharing of passwords), no web surfing at work, and no unauthorized downloads or programs on lab computers. When stepping away from the computer always lock or turn off the computer. Laptops are not to be taken out from lab unless absolutely necessary. Anyone leaving lab with one of lab's laptops must sign for possession of the laptop. No thumb drives or other removable devices should be brought into lab unless authorized.

As Lab BSO you will enforce the electronic security rules on lab. This may make you very unpopular with the lab staff, especially the ones used to recreational net surfing and youtube videos at work. However, it is necessary to prevent gaps in the electronic security of the organization.

Operational security involves background checks on all prospective employees before giving them ID's and passwords, restricting nighttime and weekend access to lab, educating lab staff on what constitutes suspicious activity, informing all lab staff of how to report and the requirement for reporting suspicious behavior, theft, etc. and requiring entry logs. If your front door has a swipe card lock, this should record which cards have been used to access the front door, obviating the need for manual logs.

As Lab BSO you have somewhat less control over the operational security. The hiring of new staff is done by the Hospital's Human Resources (HR) Department. If any prospective applicant turns out to have a significant criminal history you should ask HR to veto the hiring. The hospital's hiring is done based on HR's rules, but they should take your input seriously. In all likelihood, HR won't want a prospective employee with an arrest record, and HR will help you to prevent the hiring.

In terms of nighttime and weekend access to lab, most hospital labs are open 24 hours a day and 365 days a year. There is no way you as Lab BSO can restrict this. This situation is less likely to be a problem at a public health lab since public health labs can close at night and on weekends.

The Lab BSO is responsible for educating and training the lab staff on lab security including what constitutes suspicious activity. This includes what to report, who to report it to, etc. Suspicious activity is defined broadly as any activity that is out of the ordinary. For the purposes of reporting you only want to know about activity that could potentially indicate criminal activity. The list is quite long, but the lab staff at the minimum should be asked to report:

1. Finding the lab's front door propped open or otherwise showing evidence of an intent to compromise its integrity (scratches on the lock mechanism that were not previously noticed).
2. Finding any of lab's emergency exit doors propped open and/or with the alarm deactivated.
3. Unattended packages, backpacks, or other similar items in lab.
4. Windows found open that are normally closed.
5. Anyone paying unusual attention to the facilities and/or contents of the lab beyond a casual or professional interest.
6. Missing items in lab that cannot be accounted for, especially documents, laptops, chemicals and microbiology specimens and/or cultures.
7. Anyone loitering near the front entrance of lab and/or entering or trying to enter lab without a swipe card or visitor's pass. This includes any unauthorized individual asking to borrow a swipe card or keys for lab's doors. All lab staff are expected to question the presence of an unfamiliar person in lab and immediately report any unauthorized entry into lab.
8. Any unauthorized individual asking for passwords to lab's computer system.
9. Any unauthorized use of the lab's equipment, supplies, reagents, chemicals and/or cultures without prior approval of the lab's management.

Lab biosecurity is more important at BSL-3 and higher labs since these labs will be handling more virulent organisms compared to labs with lesser BSL capabilities. In high security labs there is typically a graded security protection. There are typically several increasing layers of security as one goes from the lab's front entrance to the areas where virulent organisms are kept. Some types of employees (delivery staff) may have swipecard access to the front door but not the BSL-2 or BSL-3 rooms. Other employees may be qualified for BSL-2 work but not BSL-3 work. Their swipecards will open the front door and BSL-2 doors, but not the BSL-3 doors, etc. The employee screening, background checks and interviews are more thorough for anyone applying for access to the more secure areas.

Typically the most sensitive areas of lab are restricted behind multiple layers of security (swipecard locks, security cameras, guards at the door checking ID badges, etc). In this setting wrongdoing by an outsider (i.e. someone without authorized access) is low and the greatest risk is from an insider (i.e someone with authorized access to your lab).

In this setting, security awareness consists of making sure all employees know how and where to report suspicious activity by another employee. The potential list is endless but at a minimum this includes: inappropriate conduct towards coworkers including inappropriate e-mails, talking about harming themself or others, unexplained absences, signs of alcohol and/or drug abuse, aggressive or violent behavior, doing work that does not correspond to official duties, working at odd hours, deception, falsifying documents, unauthorized access to computers, e-mail, etc.

30

Chapter 10 – How to read a Safety Data Sheet (SDS)

Safety Data Sheets (SDS) were formerly referred to as Material Safety Data Sheets (MSDS). These apply to chemical hazards only and do not apply to biologic or other hazards.

The Occupational Safety and Health Administration (OSHA) regulations require that for all toxic substances used in the workplace, the SDS has to be readily available in the workplace. The reference is 29 CFR § 1910.1200. This is usually accomplished by having each section of lab store a 3 ring binder with all the relevant SDS sheets in the same cabinet as that section's procedure manuals.

The SDS are typically separated into their own 3 ring binders, and not mixed in with the procedures. Make sure your lab has one SDS for each toxic substance used in the workplace. If you use bleach for cleaning, you need to have an SDS for sodium hypochlorite present in the SDS binders. At present some analyzer manufacturers are making SDS sheets for their cartridges and test kits. Make sure that for every analyzer your lab is using all relevant SDS are present in the SDS binder. The SDS sheets do not need to be signed. I have never signed an SDS binder, neither in my capacity as Lab Director nor in my capacity as Lab Biosafety Officer.

An SDS is designed as a quick reference guide containing spill control measures, health hazard information and other information for the chemical it refers to. OSHA requires the following format for all SDS:

1. Identification includes chemical name and manufacturer's name
2. Hazard identification
3. Composition and information on ingredients
4. First-aid measures
5. Fire-fighting measures
6. Accidental release measures
7. Handling and storage
8. Exposure controls and personal protection
9. Physical and chemical properties
10. Stability and reactivity
11. Toxicological information
12. Ecological information
13. Disposal considerations
14. Transport information
15. Regulatory information
16. Other information

In general, parts 1 to 13 of the SDS are self-explanatory and easy to understand. Part 14 lists the DOT and UN shipping classification of the substance. The DOT and UN regulations classify hazardous materials into the following classes:

1. Explosives
2. Gasses
3. Flammable liquid
4. Flammable solids
5. Oxidizer
6. Poisonous and Infectious substances
7. Radioactive material

8. Corrosive material
9. Miscellaneous hazardous material

Some of these classes are broken down into divisions. For example class 6 is broken down into 6.1 Poisonous materials and 6.2 Infectious substances (etiologic agents).

As a Lab BSO you don't really need to know all the codes in parts 14 through 16 of the SDS. These codes mainly deal with the shipping of hazardous substances. When dealing with the disposal of hazardous chemicals, you as Lab BSO should communicate to the hospital-wide hazardous waste disposal office the name and quantity of chemical waste that needs disposing. The hospital-wide hazardous waste disposal office will instruct you on how to collect up the waste, what types of containers to use, etc. and how the waste will be given over to the hospital-wide hazardous waste disposal office for disposal.

Most hospitals have contracted outside waste disposal companies to dispose of the hospital's hazardous chemical waste. In the typical hospital, the hospital's waste disposal office collects up all the chemical waste generated throughout the hospital. This includes not only lab's waste but also any waste from radiology, housekeeping, central supply's chemical sterilizers, etc. This waste will be stored in a locked area under the control of the hospital's waste disposal office. After a sufficient quantity has built up the hospital's waste disposal office will call the outside contractor to come and collect all of the hospital's chemical waste for disposal.

On the following pages I will give the SDS for hydrochloric acid as an example. This is one of the more toxic items you will find in a clinical laboratory.

HYDROCHLORIC ACID, 36 - 38%

---

1. Product Identification

Name: Hydrochloric acid, 36-38%
Synonyms: Muriatic acid; hydrogen chloride, aqueous
CAS No.: 7647-01-0
Molecular Weight: 36.46
Chemical Formula: HCl
Manufacturer: Dauterman Chemical Industries Corporation

---

2. Hazards Identification

Pictogram(s):

Emergency Overview

POISON! DANGER! CORROSIVE. LIQUID AND MIST CAUSE SEVERE BURNS TO ALL BODY TISSUE. MAY BE FATAL IF SWALLOWED OR INHALED. INHALATION MAY CAUSE LUNG DAMAGE.

Health Rating: 3 - Severe (Poison)	Flammability Rating: 0 - None
Reactivity Rating: 1 – Slight	Contact Rating: 3 - Severe
PPE: goggles or face shield, lab coat or apron and gloves	Storage: Corrosive

----

Potential Health Effects

Inhalation: Corrosive! Inhalation of vapors can cause coughing, choking, inflammation of the nose, throat, and upper respiratory tract, and in severe cases, pulmonary edema, circulatory failure, and death.

Ingestion: Corrosive! Swallowing hydrochloric acid can cause immediate pain and burns of the mouth, throat, esophagus and gastrointestinal tract. May cause nausea, vomiting, and diarrhea. Swallowing may be fatal.

Skin Contact:
Corrosive! Can cause redness, pain, and severe skin burns. Concentrated solutions cause deep ulcers and discolor skin.

Eye Contact:
Corrosive! Vapors are irritating and may cause damage to the eyes. Contact may cause severe burns and permanent eye damage.

Chronic Exposure:
Long-term exposure to concentrated vapors may cause erosion of teeth. Long term exposures seldom occur due to the corrosive properties of the acid.

Aggravation of Pre-existing Conditions:
Persons with pre-existing skin disorders or eye disease may be more susceptible to the effects of this substance.

3. Composition/Information on Ingredients

Ingredient	CAS No	Percent	Hazardous
Hydrogen Chloride	7647-01-0	36 - 38%	Yes
Water	7732-18-5	62 - 64%	No

4. First Aid Measures

Inhalation:
Remove to fresh air. If not breathing, give artificial respiration. If breathing is difficult, give oxygen. Get medical attention immediately.

Ingestion:
DO NOT INDUCE VOMITING! Give large quantities of water or milk if available. Never give anything by mouth to an unconscious person. Get medical attention immediately.

Skin Contact:
In case of contact, immediately flush skin with plenty of water for at least 15 minutes while removing contaminated clothing and shoes. Wash clothing before reuse. Thoroughly clean shoes before reuse. Get medical attention immediately.

Eye Contact:
Immediately flush eyes with plenty of water for at least 15 minutes, lifting lower and upper eyelids occasionally. Get medical attention immediately.

5. Fire Fighting Measures

Fire:
Extreme heat or contact with metals can release flammable hydrogen gas.
Explosion:
Not considered to be an explosion hazard.
Fire Extinguishing Media:
If involved in a fire, use water spray. Neutralize with soda ash or slaked lime.
Special Information:
In the event of a fire, wear full protective clothing and NIOSH-approved self-contained breathing apparatus with full facepiece operated in the pressure demand or other positive pressure mode. Structural firefighter's protective clothing is ineffective for fires involving hydrochloric acid. Stay away from ends of tanks. Cool tanks with water spray until well after fire is out.

6. Accidental Release Measures

Ventilate area of leak or spill. Wear appropriate personal protective equipment as specified in Section 8. Isolate hazard area. Keep unnecessary and unprotected personnel from entering. Contain and recover liquid when possible. Neutralize with alkaline material (soda ash, lime), then absorb with an inert material (e. g., vermiculite, dry sand, earth), and place in a chemical waste container. Do not use combustible materials, such as saw dust. Do not flush to sewer! US Regulations (CERCLA) require reporting spills and releases to soil, water and air in excess of reportable quantities.

7. Handling and Storage

Store in a cool, dry, ventilated storage area with acid resistant floors and good drainage. Protect from physical damage. Keep out of direct sunlight and away from heat, water, and incompatible materials. Do not wash out container and use it for other purposes. When diluting, the acid should always be added slowly to water and in small amounts. Never use hot water and never add water to the acid. Water added to acid can cause uncontrolled boiling and splashing. When opening metal containers, use non-sparking tools because of the possibility of hydrogen gas being present. Containers of this material may be hazardous when empty since they retain product residues (vapors, liquid); observe all warnings and precautions listed for the product.

8. Exposure Controls/Personal Protection

Airborne Exposure Limits:
-OSHA Permissible Exposure Limit (PEL):
5 ppm Ceiling
-ACGIH Threshold Limit Value (TLV):
5 ppm Ceiling

Ventilation System:
A system of local and/or general exhaust is recommended to keep employee exposures below the Airborne Exposure Limits. Local exhaust ventilation is generally preferred because it can control the emissions of the contaminant at its source, preventing dispersion of it into the general work area. Please refer to the ACGIH document, *Industrial Ventilation, A Manual of Recommended Practices*, most recent edition, for details.

Personal Respirators (NIOSH Approved):
If the exposure limit is exceeded, a full facepiece respirator with an acid gas cartridge may be worn up to 50 times the exposure limit or the maximum use concentration specified by the appropriate regulatory agency or respirator supplier, whichever is lowest. For emergencies or instances where the exposure levels are not known, use a full-facepiece positive-pressure, air-supplied respirator. WARNING: Air purifying respirators do not protect workers in oxygen-deficient atmospheres.

Skin Protection:
Rubber or neoprene gloves and additional protection including impervious boots, apron, or coveralls, as needed in areas of unusual exposure to prevent skin contact.

Eye Protection:
Use chemical safety goggles and/or a full face shield where splashing is possible. Maintain emergency eye wash and emergency shower facilities in work area.

9. Physical and Chemical Properties

Appearance: Colorless, fuming liquid.
Odor: Pungent odor of hydrogen chloride.
Solubility: Infinite in water with slight evolution of heat.
Density: 1.18
pH: For HCL solutions: 0.0 (1.0 N), 1.0 (0.1 N), 2.0 (0.01 N)

% Volatiles by volume @ 21°C (70°F): 100
Boiling Point: 53°C (127°F) Azeotrope (20.2%) boils at 109°C (228°F)
Melting Point: -74°C (-101°F)
Vapor Density (Air=1): No information found.
Vapor Pressure (mm Hg): 190 @ 25°C (77°F)
Evaporation Rate (BuAc=1): No information found.

---

10. Stability and Reactivity

Stability:
Stable under ordinary conditions of use and storage. Containers may burst when heated.
Hazardous Decomposition Products:
When heated to decomposition, emits toxic hydrogen chloride fumes and will react with water or steam to produce heat and toxic and corrosive fumes. Thermal oxidative decomposition produces toxic chlorine fumes and explosive hydrogen gas.
Hazardous Polymerization:
Will not occur.
Incompatibilities:
A strong mineral acid, concentrated hydrochloric acid is incompatible with many substances and highly reactive with strong bases, metals, metal oxides, hydroxides, amines, carbonates and other alkaline materials. Incompatible with materials such as cyanides, sulfides, sulfites, and formaldehyde.
Conditions to Avoid:
Heat, direct sunlight

11. Toxicological Information

Inhalation rat LC50: 3124 ppm/1H; oral rabbit LD50: 900 mg/kg (Hydrochloric acid concentrated); investigated as a tumorigen, mutagen, reproductive effector.

```
--------\Cancer Lists\--------------------------------------------------------
                                      ---NTP Carcinogen---
Ingredient                            Known    Anticipated    IARC Category
-----------------------------------   -----    -----------    -------------
Hydrogen Chloride (7647-01-0)         No       No             3
Water (7732-18-5)                     No       No             None
```

12. Ecological Information

Environmental Fate:
When released into the soil, this material is not expected to biodegrade. When released into the soil, this material may leach into groundwater.
Environmental Toxicity:
This material is expected to be toxic to aquatic life.

13. Disposal Considerations

Whatever cannot be saved for recovery or recycling should be handled as hazardous waste and sent to an approved waste facility. Processing, use or contamination of this product may change the waste management options. State and local disposal regulations may differ from federal disposal regulations. Dispose of container and unused contents in accordance with federal, state and local requirements.

14. Transport Information

Domestic (Land, D.O.T.)

Proper Shipping Name: HYDROCHLORIC ACID
Hazard Class: 8
UN/NA: UN1789
Packing Group: II
Information reported for product/size: 475LB

International (Water, I.M.O.)

Proper Shipping Name: HYDROCHLORIC ACID
Hazard Class: 8
UN/NA: UN1789
Packing Group: II
Information reported for product/size: 475LB

15. Regulatory Information

```
--------\Chemical Inventory Status - Part 1\-----------------------------------
Ingredient                                        TSCA  EC   Japan  Australia
-----------------------------------------------   ----  ---  -----  ---------
Hydrogen Chloride (7647-01-0)                     Yes   Yes  Yes      Yes
Water (7732-18-5)                                 Yes   Yes  Yes      Yes


--------\Chemical Inventory Status - Part 2\-----------------------------------
                                                        --Canada--
Ingredient                                        Korea  DSL  NDSL  Phil.
-----------------------------------------------   -----  ---  ----  -----
Hydrogen Chloride (7647-01-0)                     Yes    Yes  No    Yes
Water (7732-18-5)                                 Yes    Yes  No    Yes


--------\Federal, State & International Regulations - Part 1\----------------
                                                  -SARA 302-    ------SARA 313------
Ingredient                                        RQ    TPQ    List  Chemical Catg.
-----------------------------------------------   ---   -----  ----  --------------
Hydrogen Chloride (7647-01-0)                     5000  500*   Yes        No
Water (7732-18-5)                                 No    No     No         No


--------\Federal, State & International Regulations - Part 2\----------------
                                                              -RCRA-    -TSCA-
Ingredient                                        CERCLA      261.33    8(d)
-----------------------------------------------   ------      ------    ------
Hydrogen Chloride (7647-01-0)                     5000        No        No
Water (7732-18-5)                                 No          No        No


Chemical Weapons Convention:  No      TSCA 12(b):  No     CDTA:  Yes
SARA 311/312:  Acute: Yes      Chronic: Yes  Fire: No  Pressure: No
Reactivity: No          (Mixture / Liquid)
```

---

16. Other Information

NFPA Ratings: Health: **3** Flammability: **0** Reactivity: **1**
Label Hazard Warning:
POISON! DANGER! CORROSIVE. LIQUID AND MIST CAUSE SEVERE BURNS TO ALL BODY TISSUE. MAY BE FATAL IF SWALLOWED OR INHALED. INHALATION MAY CAUSE LUNG DAMAGE.
Label Precautions:
Do not get in eyes, on skin, or on clothing.
Do not breathe vapor or mist.
Use only with adequate ventilation.
Wash thoroughly after handling.
Store in a tightly closed container.
Remove and wash contaminated clothing promptly.
Label First Aid:
In case of contact, immediately flush eyes or skin with plenty of water for at least 15 minutes while removing contaminated clothing and shoes. Wash clothing before reuse. If swallowed, DO NOT INDUCE VOMITING. Give large quantities of water. Never give anything by mouth to an unconscious person. If inhaled, remove to fresh air. If not breathing, give artificial respiration. If breathing is difficult, give oxygen. In all cases get medical attention immediately.
Product Use:
Laboratory Reagent.
Revision Information:
SDS Section(s) changed since last revision of document include: 16.

Chapter 11 – Responding to spills, accidents, disasters, etc.

Minor spills in lab are relatively common. Most of these will involve relatively nontoxic materials in small quantities, for example formalin spills in histology section, spilled acid alcohol for Fite staining in Microbiology section, etc. Make sure you have spill kits in lab so you can throw the towels down on the spill. If the spill is too large to be covered by all the towels in lab's spill kits, you may have to call in the hospital-wide hazard responders.

I have not seen more serious accidents happening in my own workplace. The best advice is to make sure all the SDS are in an easy to retrieve binder, so that you can find information on how to deal with the problem quickly when it happens.

OSHA requires a policy for dealing with bloodborne pathogens. The reference is 29 CFR § 1910.1030. Make sure all lab staff are familiar with the needlestick policy. If a needlestick happens, some of the HIV prophylaxis protocols call for the medications to be given within 72 hours of the needlestick. You will need to deal with this situation immediately when it happens, and there won't be time to figure things out after the fact.

To briefly summarize the typical needlestick policy, wash needlesticks with soap and water. If no soap is available use alcohol based hand rubs. Report the incident to your supervisor then immediately seek medical treatment. The source patient for the needlestick (if known) should be tested for HIV, Hepatitis B and Hepatitis C. The healthcare worker stuck by the needle will typically be started on post-exposure prophylaxis before the test results are available for the source patient. If the testing of the source patient comes back as negative the post-exposure prophylaxis may be discontinued.

Make sure all lab staff get their Employee Health Clearance on time. Typically this clearance entails PPD skin testing for tuberculosis. Follow up with the Employee Health office at least monthly to make sure there are no lab staff delinquent in their PPD's. If there is a PPD converter in lab you will need to investigate to determine if it was a laboratory acquired infection.

The hospital lab where I work also doubles as a public health lab. This means we will rarely receive environmental specimens for testing. The most common situation where an emergency response is requested is when white powder is found at the airport. When the local airport finds a white power, their policies call for the white powder to be tested for drugs of abuse. The airport has its own test kits for drugs of abuse, so the local hospital/public health lab is not involved at this point. If the powder tests positive for drugs of abuse the airport will not need further testing of the powder.

If the white powder tests negative for drugs of abuse, the airport will insist on immediate testing of the powder to rule out anthrax. The airport does not have any capability to test for anthrax on site and at one time insisted on calling the Lab Biosafety Officer to come and collect up the white powder and have it tested for anthrax. The problem is that most cargo flights into the airport arrive between 2AM and 4AM. This generated multiple late night calls to the former Lab Biosafety Officer. According to the former Lab Biosafety Officer, this is one of the main reasons he quit the job. He has young children and couldn't take the late night calls from the airport. The former Lab BSO had been asking the airport to stop calling him at night. The hospital/public health lab can't do anthrax testing and sends the specimens out. The specimens can wait at the airport until morning, since they could not be packaged for send-out until the lab's day staff comes in at 7AM.

In the time I have been Lab BSO I have not had any nighttime calls from the airport. I assume the airport must have changed its procedures for dealing with white powder. From attending a bioterrorism meeting in mid-2017, it is my understanding that the current routing of a white powder is from the place where it is found (the airport) to the local FBI office to the remote testing site. This means the local hospital/public health lab is not currently party to the transport of the specimen. I am grateful for this, since I would not want to get lots of nighttime calls from the airport.

The airport's calls have all been false alarms. All of their white powders tested negative for anthrax. The airport had kept outdated procedures in its procedure manuals for an extended length of time.

Every time there is a significant accident in lab it must be documented. The lab must report to OSHA all accidents, spills, chemical exposures, injuries and biologic exposures. An incident report should be generated for any untoward event in these categories, so as to be able to keep track of any occurrences.

Most biosafety manuals require that significant accidents in lab must be reported by the Lab BSO to the Lab Director, Risk Manager and/or hospital CEO. If the hospital has an Institutional Biosafety Committee (IBC) the accident should be reported to the IBC as well.

After any accident you as Lab BSO will need to investigate the specifics. How and why did the accident occur? What contributed to the accident? How can the lab be made safer to prevent recurrence of this type of accident?

Make sure all risks have been addressed. A significant accident typically results from multiple things going wrong at the same time. The usual approach is the plan, do, check, act (PDCA) cycle used for continuous quality improvement. This is also known as the Deming cycle and the Shewhart cycle.

The four steps of the plan, do, check, act cycle are:

1. Plan - examine an existing process and try to determine ways it can be improved upon.
2. Do – small changes are put in place. This is a small scale test of the planned solution to determine how effective it is.
3. Check – in this step you check to see how effective the small scale changes are.
4. Act – if the small scale changes are effective, put the changes in place on a larger scale. If the small scale changes are not effective, start over from the planning stage.

For example, let me give the hypothetical scenario of a formalin spill. In this scenario, the 10% formalin is dispensed from a 5 gallon container into cups. The lab tech dispensing the formalin notices that the lids are ill-fitting on the cups but continues to fill them and gives them to the Operating Room (O.R.). Later that day, several specimens are brought back from O.R. with the formalin slopping out of the container into the biohazard bag. One of these bags spills its formalin onto the histology room floor when opened by the histotech.

As with most accidents multiple things went wrong. The histotech did not stop after noticing the formalin container lids are ill-fitting. The histotech should be reminded of the policy that any defective items in lab should be reported and replaced immediately. The O.R. also did not notice that the formalin container lids are ill-fitting. The O.R. likewise should be reminded not to use formalin containers if the lids don't fit the container properly. The histotech opened a biohazard bag containing formalin over the floor and not inside the histology hood. The histotech should be reminded of the policy that that anything containing formalin should only be opened inside the histology hood.

After putting mitigations in place (replace defective formalin containers, educate the histotech, etc.) the next step is to check that the mitigations have been effective. Once per week or once per month walk into the histology section and check that the lids are tight on that day's formalin containers. If the lids are still ill-fitting additional work needs to be done – consider buying the containers from a different vendor. Consider asking O.R. to send the specimens to lab without formalin and adding the formalin to the specimens in lab, etc.

The above scenario follows the plan, do, check, act cycle. The planning phase is examining the processes involved to see where the failure occurred. The do phase is the stage where the defective formalin containers are replaced and the histotech is educated. The check phase occurs when you follow up in histology to make sure the lids are secure on the formalin containers. The act phase is when you decide that the fix you put in place works, and the fix is made permanent (no more defective formalin containers allowed in laboratory).

The literature indicates that as a Lab BSO you should take a root cause analysis (RCA) approach to accidents and incidents in lab. As the name implies, an RCA tries to identify the root cause of the incident. In the example above the root cause of the problem was that the lids were ill-fitting on the formalin containers.

In order to do an RCA properly you must examine the entire system involved. For the example above, you must examine the entire process of formalin use: The formalin arrives in lab as gallon size containers of 100% formalin. The 100% formalin is mixed down to 10% formalin in a five gallon container under the histology hood. From there the 10% formalin is dispensed into 100ml, 250ml and liter size containers which are given to the O.R. During surgery the O.R. collects specimens into the formalin containers. For each specimen the O.R. is supposed to check the container lid to ensure the lid is tight and then put the container in a biohazard bag. The specimens are sent to lab and processed under the histology hood.

The specimens are then stored in a specimen cabinet until three weeks after the histology report is ready. The specimen containers are then moved back under the histology hood where the specimens are separated from the formalin. The tissue specimens are put in red biohazard trash bags and given over to housekeeping to incinerate in the hospital incinerator. The waste formalin is stored in histology until 5 gallons accumulates at which time it is disposed by the hospital-wide hazardous waste disposal office. The empty specimen containers are put in red biohazard trash bags for disposal with lab's other red bag trash.

When doing an RCA it is not sufficient to take the easy way out and say "it's all the histotechnologist's fault". This would not be considered an adequate RCA.

Another technique for doing an RCA involves repeatedly asking "Why?" until one comes to the root cause of the problem. This technique is mentioned in the COLA literature. In my experience, there is no way to know when you have reached the root cause and it is time to stop asking "Why?". Instead, one could ask "Why?" forever. I prefer the systematic approach given above. It has a defined start, systematic way of looking at the problem, and a defined end point.

All work done must be documented including the accident investigation and mitigations put in place after the accident. This documentation is usually kept with the incident report for the accident. This is typically stored in the hospital Risk Manager's office.

OSHA does not specifically require fire drills, but recommends that they should be conducted at least annually. Most hospitals I have worked at have annual fire drills and disaster drills. These can be a fun diversion from the routine work at hand. The simplest disaster drill consists of herding all the lab staff out into a corridor deemed to be safe from tornadoes. I have been to much more elaborate drills, including mass casualty disaster drills conducted as a joint exercise between the hospital and airport. In these drills actors were painted with red paint at the airport to simulate blood then driven by ambulance to the hospital. One fire drill I went to had a "live fire" exercise in which the trainers took the trainees into the parking lot, set fire to a barrel full of newspapers and the trainees one-by-one had to put out the fire using a fire extinguisher. Most public health labs will additionally have annual drills for Pandemic Influenza, Ebola, accidental release of organisms, bioterrorism, etc.

All labs are required to have a disaster plan. Most of the lab disaster plans I have seen center on recalling staff, stockpiling enough reagents and supplies to meet an anticipated surge in lab testing after the disaster, stockpiling blood units in Blood Bank, limiting testing to STAT testing (no routine testing until the disaster is over), stockpiling food and water for the hospital staff and patients, stockpiling fuel for the generator, leadership and chain of command delegation (Incident Commander takes over from Hospital Administrator until the disaster is over), increased security presence, communication using satellite telephones, making back-up copies of lab records, plans for shutdown of the lab with evacuation of the building, plans to relocate testing to a different site, etc. The disaster plan is usually kept in the laboratory's general procedure manual. Everyone in lab is required to read and sign the disaster plan as well as the rest of the lab's general procedure manual.

After a major disaster, the most important tasks relate to continuity of the lab's operations. The lab's goal after a community-wide disaster is to continue with the testing and preserve lab records to the extent possible.

In my 28 years in Pathology and Lab Medicine I have been present for four disasters that I consider to be major disasters – the August 6, 1997 crash of Korean Airlines flight 801 on Guam, Typhoon Pongsona on December 8, 2002 on Guam, Typhoon Soudelor on August 2, 2015 on Saipan and Typhoon Yutu on October 24, 2018 on Saipan. In each of these disasters, some the above list of preparations helped somewhat. Most of the above list of preparations would prove unnecessary; while other, unexpected problems cropped up. In other words, in this setting you need to be flexible and find workarounds for problems as they appear.

The only real mass casualty disaster I have attended to was the August 6, 1997 crash of Korean Airlines flight 801. It went down on Guam with 254 people aboard a little after 1AM. At the time of the crash, I was one of three Pathologists working at Guam Memorial Hospital (GMH) and there was a military pathologist at the Guam Naval Hospital. The Guam Medical Examiner was on vacation and unavailable at the time of the crash. At about 3AM I was paged to come in to work at GMH and stationed at the Blood Bank. The other GMH Pathologists were assigned to the site of the crash and tasked with body identification and body recovery. The Navy pathologist was assigned to work at the Naval Hospital Blood Bank to help mobilize their frozen blood supply.

In the first 24 hours after the crash, GMH Blood Bank drew close to 100 blood donors. I did the donor screening and most of the donor interviews. There were 6 lab techs that drew the donors. We all worked non-stop at a frantic pace the first 24 hours after the crash. If anyone told me that it would be possible to do that much work in 24 hours I would not have believed them.

In this particular disaster there were few survivors. Only about 28 of the 254 people on board the aircraft survived. There was little surge in test volume after the crash, since there were few survivors. The main problem for lab related to morgue capacity. The number of deceased remains recovered from the crash far exceeded the morgue capacity of all local hospitals, the Medical Examiner's and all local funeral homes combined. The body recovery and identification occurred over several weeks on the Navy Base. The first intact 75 bodies were brought to a Navy refrigerated storage location and later the bodies and body parts were placed in refrigerator trucks. Many of the remains were fragmented which made identification difficult. In many cases identification was by DNA matching to surviving relatives. In the late 1990s this type of testing took months to complete. Most of the remains were stored in refrigerated trailers until they could be identified and buried.

Here is a picture of the service pin I received from the Government of Guam for my work done after the crash of KAL flight 801.

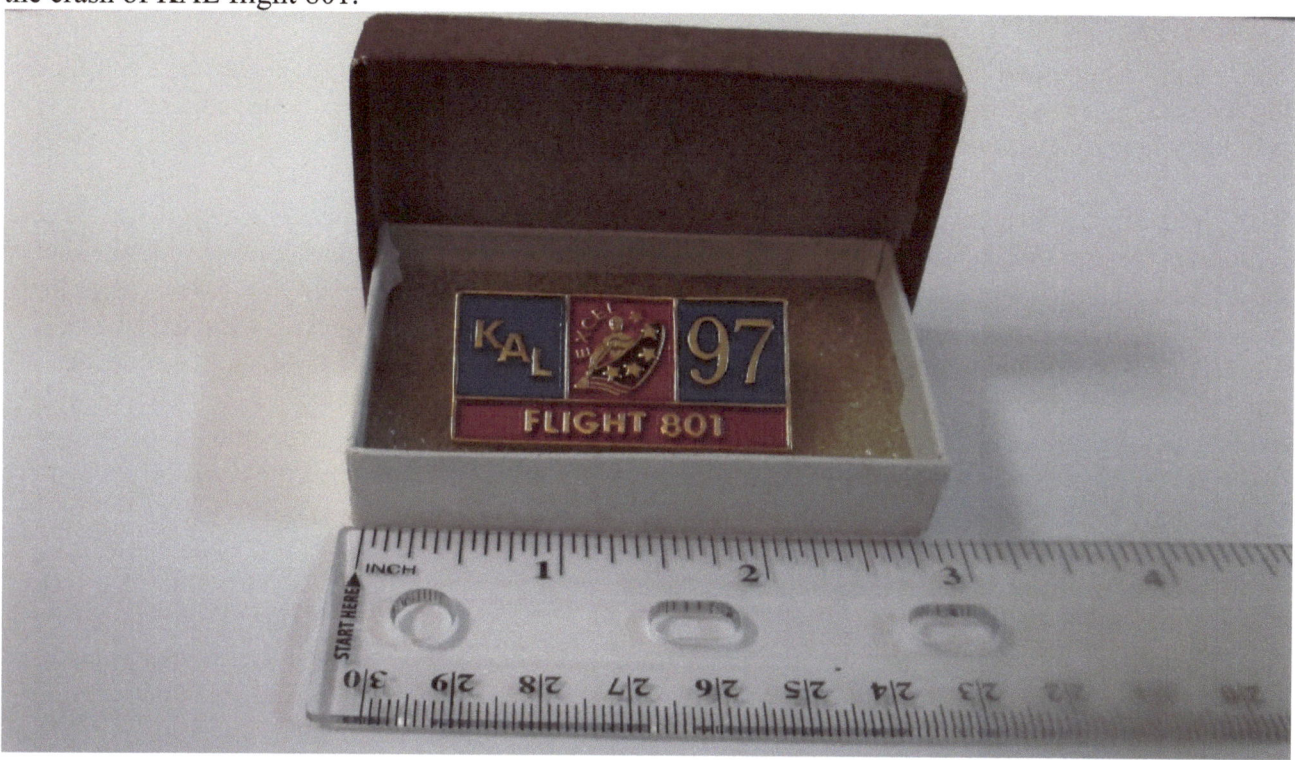

I was on Guam at the time of Typhoon Pongsona which hit December 8, 2002. This storm would have been considered a category 4 hurricane if it was on the Atlantic; however, different terminology is used in the Pacific. It was not a mass casualty disaster on Guam, there were no direct fatalities. However, it did extensive damage to the infrastructure. There was no running water for weeks, no electric power for months, and no gasoline at the gas stations for about 2 weeks. The roads were impassable for several days until the debris was removed from the roadways. The telecommunication system also failed with almost all telephone poles and lines downed by the storm. Cellphones were restored in a few days but landlines and internet service took months to restore. Once cellphones came back up we were placing supply/reagent orders using cellphones until the landlines and internet service were restored.

At the time of the storm, the electric grid failed and the hospital went on generator power. The hospital's generator failed in the storm and the hospital was without electric power for about 12 hours. Testing had to be suspended while there was no electric power, but resumed after the generator was restored. Some parts of lab had flooded from rainwater permeating a damaged roof. This was relatively easy to clean up with no structural damage to the interior of the lab from the storm.

It took weeks to restore the connection to the local electric utility, and during this time the lab was running on the hospital's generator power. Generator power is subject to frequent spikes and outages, which disrupted lab's operations. It is imperative to have all of lab's critical equipment on an Uninterruptible Power Supply (UPS). Any equipment that was not on a UPS would be damaged or destroyed by the power outages and power spikes in this situation.

Under these conditions, the hospital-wide computer system is very problematic. It tends to crash with each power out and power spike. If the hospital-wide computer system is going to be down for an extended length of time, the lab will have to revert to printing paper lab results and hand delivering the paper lab results to the wards, ER, clinics, etc. In this situation, make sure to inventory your stock of printer paper and toner cartridges, as you will be using these up much faster than usual. You may also need to ask for additional secretarial help to hand deliver all the paper lab reports.

The hospital's generator was not powerful enough to fully run the air conditioning system. Several lab instruments began to give overheat alarms. These instruments had their covers removed, and were cooled by fan while still continuing with the testing.

In the immediate aftermath of the storm, the main problems related to resupply. The airport was closed for about 2 weeks after the storm, and by the time it reopened the lab was running low or running out of most essential items. Some local vendors had their businesses completely destroyed, or had major loss of inventory in the storm. Most local vendors were unable to open their businesses most days because of lack of electric power to run the vendor's computers and inventory system and lack of employees reporting to work. The reason most employees were not reporting to work was because of impassable roads, lack of gasoline at the gas stations making commuting impossible, the large number of damaged/destroyed houses were a more immediate priority than work, and the employees needed to secure food and drinkable water for themselves and their families.

At the start of each working day, the first thing I would do is to check what is working and what is not working in lab, check which testing is available and which testing is suspended due to reagent outage. Next I would inventory all critical supplies in lab, then call all the vendors to see which vendors would be able to open for business that day and which would not. Each time a vendor was able to open, I would ask the hospital's Materials Management Office to buy as much lab-related inventory as possible, since there was no way of knowing if that vendor would be able to open their business again in the short term.

FEMA staff did not arrive at the hospital until about 2 days after the storm passed. They were not present in large numbers until at least 5 days after the storm. Their first priority was ensuring adequate supplies, continuous electric power and potable water for the hospital. Immediately after arriving, the FEMA staff will typically call a meeting with all hospital department heads and separate meetings with hospital administration. Be prepared to give the FEMA staff a copy of your inventory lists and list of reagent shortages/outages the first time you meet with them.

Many of the businesses that were destroyed in the storm never reopened. Instead the owners collected the insurance checks and moved to the US Mainland, relocating their businesses. The reduced number of vendors available after the storm affected procurement.

It is particularly important to keep the microbiology testing functional after a disaster. The conditions after a disaster are conducive to epidemics - large numbers of people crowded into shelters, lack of running water for basic hygiene, lack of basic sanitation, lack of drinkable water, etc.

46

Staffing was an issue after Pongsona. In the immediate aftermath of the storm most lab staff were not able to report to work due to impassable roads, no gas at the gas stations, their homes were damaged or destroyed, they needed to secure food and drinkable water for themselves and their families, etc. Lack of gasoline was a greater problem for lab staff that lived further from the hospital as they would need more gas to commute to work. A rule was put in place that each staff member must work until relieved (i.e until their replacement arrived to work). This resulted in many lab staff having to work two consecutive 8-hour shifts. We tried to arrange things so that no one had three consecutive 8-hour shifts, but this was unavoidable in a few cases.

On a personal level, Guam after Pongsona resembled a death trap. There was little access to food or drinkable water. The hospital reserved its food and water for the patients and did not give any food or water to the employees. There was no way out - the airport was closed. At the time the storm hit, I had about two week's supply of food and water in my apartment. For the first two weeks after Pongsona, I was using up the food and water in my apartment. The next several weeks, it was catch as catch can in a time when stores would reopen, quickly sell out of all food and water, then close again until they could restock. During most of this time frame I had less than a 2 day supply of food and drinkable water available. FEMA eventually provided Meal Ready to Eat (MRE) rations to the hospital staff. This was too little, too late, and the MRE were not very appetizing anyhow. The situation would improve later on as more stores restocked and reopened.

The airport cleared its runway of debris and reopened for flights about 2 weeks after the storm. After the airport reopened there was a mass exodus. I can't count how many going-away parties I went to in the next 3 months. I am guessing about 10% to 20% of the population left and never returned. A few lab staff quit and moved away, but the test volume was down due to mass exodus, so this pretty much evened out. Things did not reach a more normal state until about 3 to 6 months after the storm.

I was on Saipan at the time of Typhoon Yutu which hit October 24, 2018. It was the equivalent of a strong Category 5 hurricane on the Atlantic. This storm hit with sustained winds of 180 MPH making it the second strongest landfalling tropical cyclone in the history of the US and the sixth strongest landfalling tropical cyclone in the history of the world. It did considerably more damage than any prior typhoon I have seen. The usual post-disaster problems of protracted airport closure and staff unable to report to work occurred. The hospital did not lose power or water. However, as is typical of a major disaster there were protracted power outages in the community. The recovery of the water system and gas at the gas stations was faster than for previous typhoons.

After this disaster, the main problem from lab's perspective related to the airport closure. The airport was not able to open for inbound traffic for about a week after the storm. Several shipments were delayed including our hematology controls. The hematology controls arrived warm with the ice packs melted. We contacted the vendor's technical service department and they said to test the controls. We ran 20 repeat runs of the received warm controls and the results were acceptable. The technical service department said to use the received warm controls. Even so, I insisted on a replacement and the vendor replaced the received warm controls with a new shipment of controls which were received cold.

Another problem after Typhoon Yutu involved shipping of specimens off from Saipan for reference testing. For example, the lab receives numerous specimens for tuberculosis testing, but only has a BSL-2 capability. All specimens for tuberculosis culture must be sent out and the nearest reference lab offering tuberculosis culture is in Hawaii. The airport remained closed for outbound shipments for about two weeks after the storm. After about 2 weeks, I received notice from the hospital's preparedness office that the airport had reopened for outbound shipments.

Over the course of the next week, all local couriers were refusing to accept outbound shipments as they had not received the "all clear" from the airport to send outbound shipments. It took several phone calls, meetings and E-mail to inform all the couriers that the airport was open for outbound shipments. In that time we had many specimens waiting for shipping for send-out reference testing. For specimens with short stability (tuberculosis culture, newborn screening, etc.) we informed the patients that we could not collect the specimens due to shipping issues and we would call them back for specimen collection when we are able to ship the specimens out for testing.

In this disaster, my car 's rear window was broken by flying debris. However, there was no damage to my apartment. My car insurance was with a local company whose office was almost completely destroyed by the storm. One's car insurance is only as good as the company providing it. There is no way to file a claim with a defunct insurance company. Next, I tried filing with FEMA for the broken car window.

From what I have been told, FEMA only reimburses if there is damage to the house or the car is undrivable. See below. I was told that my damage did not meet FEMA's criteria because my house was undamaged and the car was still drivable with the rear window broken. FEMA did not reimburse my $650 out of pocket expense for the car window repair. Instead, FEMA referred me to the Small Business Administration (SBA) for a loan. See below explanation:

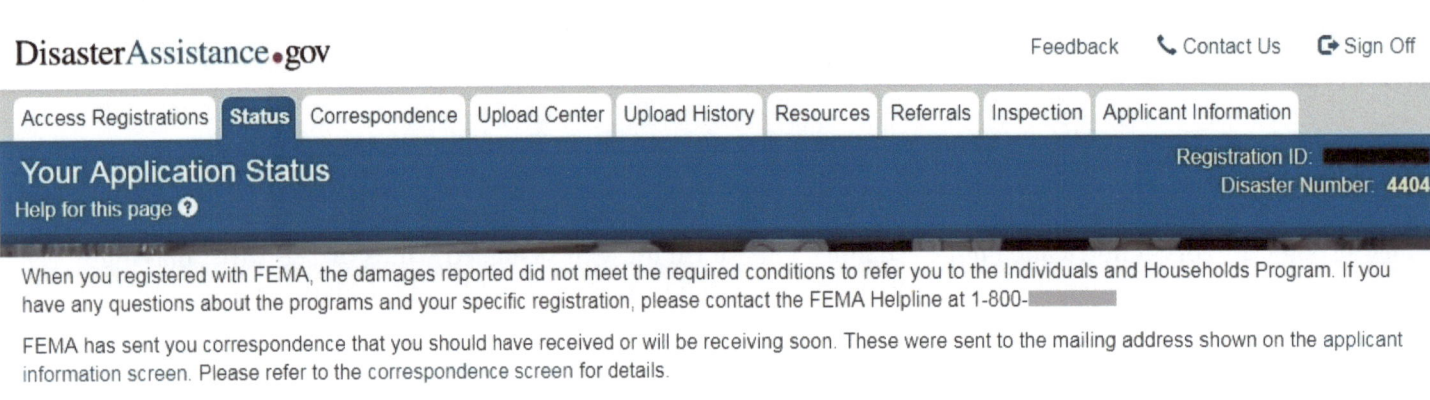

I waited in line two hours to meet with an SBA representative at a Disaster Recovery Center on Saipan.

48

The SBA offered to loan up to the $650 loss at a low interest rate. They said that the loan could not be for more than the $650 damage incurred by the storm. This would have involved filling out paperwork, scheduling an SBA inspector to look at the broken car window, etc. The SBA representative said that for small dollar amount loans, the loan typically has to be paid back within a year or two. By the time I met with the SBA representative I had already paid the $650 out of pocket to replace the broken rear car window. I was still in good financial condition without the $650 and did not bother to file for the SBA loan.

I spent hours waiting in line at the FEMA and SBA offices while filing the claim for the broken car window and had the opportunity to speak with several of their staff. The FEMA and SBA staff were impressed with the extent of the damage from Typhoon Yutu, This was the worst storm I have ever seen, and some of the FEMA and SBA people had never seen a category 5 tropical cyclone either. You know things are bad when the FEMA and SBA staff are impressed with the destruction.

At least this time around I got more Meals Ready to Eat (MRE) from FEMA and did not lose as much weight (215 pounds at the time of Typhoon Yutu down to 203 pounds one month later) compared to prior typhoons. I also got some free Disaster Response Training:

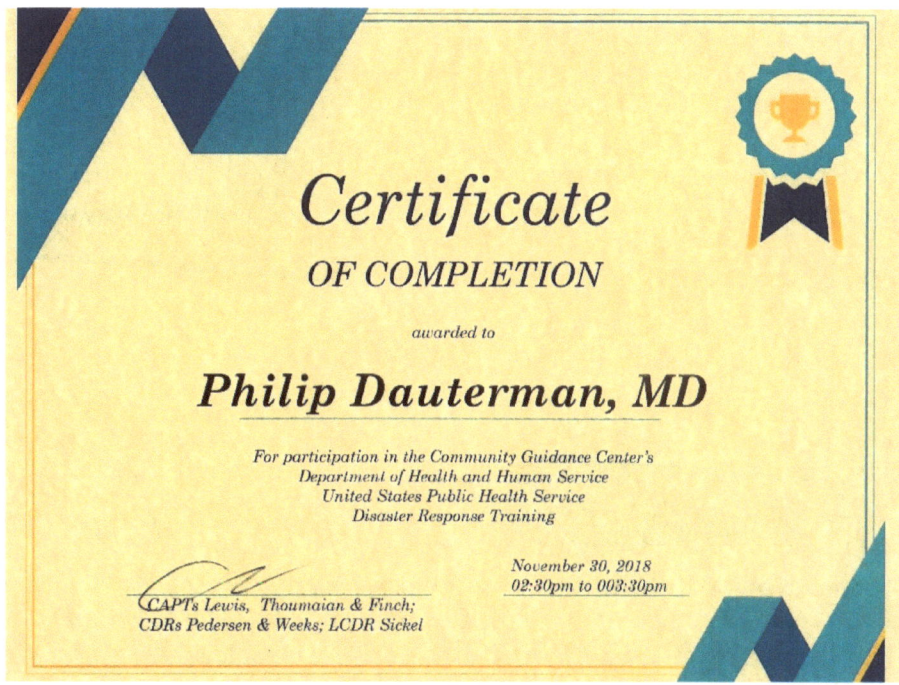

After the disaster was over, the hospital I work for asked me to list the additional work done above and beyond my usual duties. The response was:

1. Ensure the lab has adequate supplies by providing inventory lists to Incident Command (IC) and arranging with IC for alternate routes for supply shipments.
2. Ensure 24/7 coverage of laboratory as several lab staff were not able to report to work due to damaged/destroyed homes. The work schedules were increased for the staff that were able to report to work.
3. Ensure continuity of lab's operations, including outbound shipping of specimens for off-site reference lab testing. Several specimens were delayed in shipping out due to problems at the airport. This was resolved with coordination from IC.

About 3 months after the storm, the landlord of the apartment building where I live sent notice that all units in the building would have a rent increase of $50/month. This letter stated that essentially all businesses on Saipan had incurred significant expenses from repairs after the storm. All businesses on Saipan were passing the costs onto the customer in the form of higher rates. The landlord would have higher costs for all goods and services for the foreseeable future and had no choice but to raise the rent to offset the higher maintenance expenses. In this setting, I paid the higher rent without questioning. The apartment building where I live is made of concrete and survived the storm intact. I am guessing about 15% of the houses on Saipan were completely destroyed (roof gone, walls gone, nothing left but debris) and another 30% were severely damaged (roof gone, walls still standing). With large numbers of displaced people looking for shelter one needs to stay on good terms with one's landlord. Even the lab staff were not spared from the dislocation. Four of seventeen lab staff lost their homes in the storm and were living in temporary housing arrangements for months after the storm.

In closing, I would like to thank the lab and hospital staff that reported to work during and after the disasters listed above. Many of the lab staff were working despite significant personal hardships including damaged or destroyed homes yet they continued to report to work on schedule. This shows the dedication and determination of everyone in lab. It is an honor to be a part of this.

Chapter 12 – Disinfection, high level disinfection, sterilization and autoclaves

Disinfection, decontamination and sanitization are largely synonymous. The intent is to render a contaminated item safe enough to handle. Disinfection kills all nonsporulated microorganisms and most spores.

Sterilization kills ALL microorganisms on an inanimate object, even the spores. Spores are particularly difficult to kill, and the typical disinfection does not kill all the spores.

High Level Disinfection kills all nonsporulated organisms and almost all spores. This is intermediate between an ordinary disinfection and a sterilization. Regulations require the Operating Room (O.R.) to perform high level disinfection is many settings (for example moving laryngoscope blades and some endoscopes from one patient to another). There are no regulatory requirements to use high level disinfection in lab. As far as lab is concerned something is either sterile or it isn't. Thus for lab's purposes disinfection is the same as high level disinfection. High level disinfection is not used in any laboratory I am familiar with. However, you will still need to know the terminology as the O.R. staff will use this terminology repeatedly in your biosafety meetings.

Disinfection is used when it is not necessary to kill all the microorganisms on a surface. For example, at the end of each day the interior of the BSC cabinet is disinfected with bleach or alcohol. There is no need for sterilization of the BSC's interior surfaces. On the other hand, Microbiology Petri agar plates must be absolutely sterile before use so as to avoid false positive test results.

In my experience the most common disinfectants used in hospital labs are:

Bleach (sodium hypochlorite solution) – the most popular lab disinfectant, it is relatively nontoxic to humans but highly lethal to microorganisms. Disadvantages include its tendency to discolor and corrode metals. Disposal of bleach is not an issue; it can be mixed with water and disposed down the drain.

Alcohol (isopropyl alcohol or ethanol) – the second most popular lab disinfectant, it is relatively nontoxic to humans but highly lethal to microorganisms. The disadvantage of alcohols is their high flammability. Disposal of waste/unused alcohol is an issue due to the flammability.

Iodine solutions (for example betadine) – used as a skin swab prior to drawing blood samples in phlebotomy. It can also be used as a lab disinfectant but this is uncommon. It is relatively nontoxic to humans but highly lethal to microorganisms. However, it tends to leave messy residues on surfaces, and has an odor. Disposal of used betadine swabs is not an issue, they can go in red bag or white bag trash.

Hydrogen peroxide – Used in the clinical setting to disinfect skin wounds, injuries, etc. I have heard of this being used as a disinfectant in labs, but this is uncommon. It is relatively nontoxic to humans but is less effective at killing microorganisms (requires longer contact times) as compared to bleach or alcohols. Disposal of 3% hydrogen peroxide is not an issue; it can go down the sink undiluted.

Formaldehyde – used in histology section for preserving tissue. It is possible to use this as a lab disinfectant, but this is hardly ever done. The main problem with formaldehyde solutions is their strong odor. Formaldehyde is considered a HazMat chemical. It requires PPE for use as a disinfectant and HazMat disposal for any waste/unused amount.

Other disinfectants including phenol, peracetic acid, ortho-phthalaldehyde (OPA), quaternary ammonium compounds, etc. are on the market. These have a small market share in the US. Be careful with these as some of them (for example phenol) are highly toxic to humans. If you are going to be using phenol as a disinfectant, you will need to dress up in PPE (face shield, apron and gloves). It doesn't make sense to dress up in this much PPE when you can disinfect using bleach or alcohol wearing only gloves.

Each of the various disinfectants listed above will have a required minimum contact time. Make sure the lab staff are following the manufacturer's directions for use of the disinfectant, especially the contact time. For some of the above disinfectants the contact time is prolonged, several minutes or more, and the lab staff won't want to wait this long before moving on to their next task. Another caveat is to make sure the disinfectant you are using is compatible with the equipment you are using it on. As mentioned above, bleach tends to corrode metal. If this presents a problem for your equipment, use a different disinfectant.

As mentioned above, sterilization kills ALL microorganisms. This is needed for anything that must be completely sterile (for example making Microbiology Petri agar plates). Sterilizers have two uses in lab. First, they can be used to sterilize supplies and equipment prior to use, typically in the Microbiology section of lab. Second, they can be used to sterilize waste prior to disposal.

Sterilizers either use chemicals or steam for sterilization. Steam sterilizers are called autoclaves. In clinical labs autoclaves are commonplace whereas chemical sterilizers are not often used. The chemicals used in chemical sterilizers are typically toxic; thus, chemical sterilizers present more problems than autoclaves due to their need for toxic chemicals, risk of operator exposure to the chemicals and need to dispose of those chemicals when done sterilizing.

There are some situations where chemical sterilization can't be avoided. If the item to be sterilized can't survive the heat, pressure or moisture of an autoclave, the item can't be autoclaved. If the item needs to be sterilized you will need to have a chemical sterilizer. If you get a chemical sterilizer you will need a supply of chemicals, disposal of waste chemicals, a supply of chemical indicator autoclave tape, biological indicators for chemical sterilization, etc.

From a cost and supply perspective, the operation of a chemical sterilizer is much more expensive and difficult than an autoclave. It is much easier to select all your equipment and supplies to be autoclave safe. When you are selecting new equipment and supplies, especially for the microbiology section, ensure that they are autoclavable to the extent possible. For almost all items in lab (pipette tips, dispensers, thermometers, etc.) you can find some manufacturer somewhere that is making an autoclave safe version. Try to buy autoclave safe items to the extent you can unless you want to have all the headaches of dealing with a chemical sterilizer.

Autoclaves use either gravity or vacuum to perfuse the chamber with steam. In most autoclaves steam is pumped into the chamber and perfuses the contents by gravity. In some autoclaves the air is pumped out of the chamber creating a vacuum before the steam is introduced and/or pulses of steam and vacuum are used.

Prior to getting an autoclave, my lab's red bag waste flow was collected by housekeeping from the red trash cans and brought downstairs to the hospital-wide autoclave for sterilization then disposal. Someone objected that lab's red bag trash included Microbiology's used culture plates which contained live cultures. It was decided that lab must get its own autoclave to sterilize these used Microbiology Petri agar plates before the plates leave the laboratory.

My lab bought a midsize tabletop autoclave and installed it in a room adjacent to Microbiology. It came from the manufacturer pre-programmed with two settings:

1. 121°C (250°F) held for 30 minutes under pressure of 15 PSI
2. 132°C (270°F) held for 10 minutes under pressure of 30 PSI

These are the two most commonly used settings on a steam autoclave using gravity to perfuse the chamber. If you are autoclaving a large load of waste (over 10 pounds) you should set the sterilization time to at least double the time given above (i.e. at least 60 minutes at 250°F or 20 minutes at 270°F). Use a slow exhaust cycle when autoclaving liquids to minimize boiling over. The cycle time will typically be shorter for an autoclave using vacuum to perfuse the chamber. In an autoclave using vacuum, the vacuum rapidly draws steam into areas that would be slow to perfuse using gravity.

Some autoclaves use temperatures above 270°F for shorter durations. This is referred to as "flash sterilization". This is used in O.R.'s where equipment must go rapidly from patient to patient. Flash sterilization is hardly ever done in lab since you don't typically need to sterilize trash quickly.

The typical temperature cycle for a steam autoclave using gravity perfusion is depicted below:

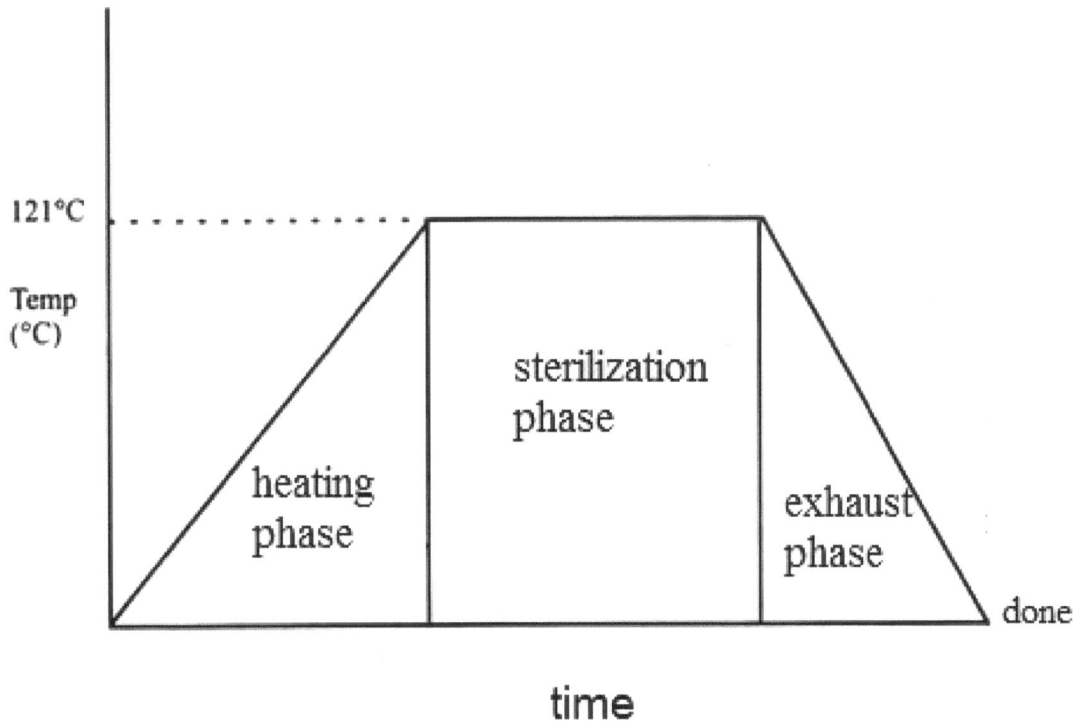

The typical steam autoclave allows you to change the settings. You can increase or decrease the temperature, sterilization time, exhaust time, etc. Be VERY careful when decreasing the time or temperature of sterilization. If you do not meet the minimum sterilization time and/or temperature, the waste could come out of the autoclave still contaminated and potentially infectious.

As a final caveat, the autoclave and everything in it will be dangerously hot at the end of the cycle. Thermal protective PPE (autoclave gloves, etc.) must be worn when removing items from the autoclave.

My lab's autoclave came from the manufacturer pre-programmed with the 270°F for 10 minutes setting. Here's what it did to the autoclave trash bag:

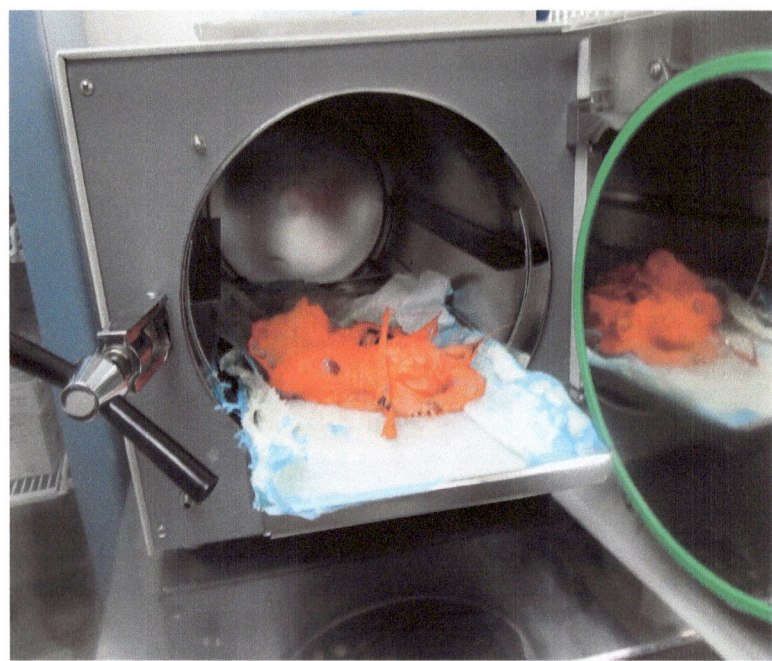

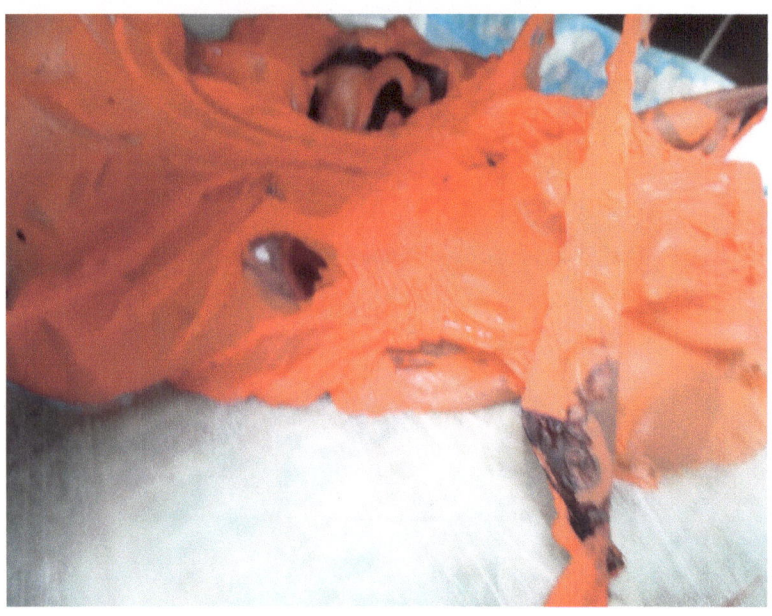

The first test run with lab's new autoclave was quite a disaster. The plastic bag melted inside the autoclave and the contents of liquefied agar dripped out. Luckily the test run involved expired agar plates that had never been used. It took housekeeping more than an hour to clean out the mess on the inside of the autoclave.

On closer inspection the fine print on the autoclave bags indicates they are only to be used up to 250°F. We changed our autoclave to the lower, longer sterilization setting and this problem did not recur. The autoclave bags were able to survive the 250°F autoclaving intact without melting or tearing holes. I also obtained a metal pan to put underneath the autoclave bag to catch any leaking.

Here is a picture of my lab's next test run. This was a successful run:

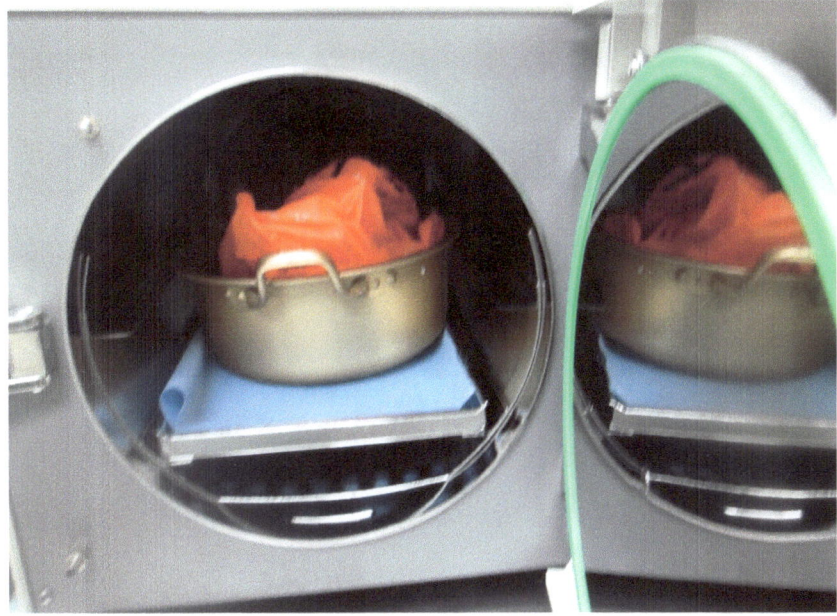

The plan going forward is that lab will put the used Microbiology Petri agar plates into red bags, loosely seal them with color changing autoclave tape, autoclave them, then put the autoclaved bags into the red trash can. Housekeeping will pick these up with the other red bag trash, take them to the hospital wide autoclave and they will be autoclaved again. This will ensure sterility of the waste leaving lab.

Autoclaving waste requires the use of sterilization indicators. Indicators of sterilization are either chemical (color changing tape, cards, kits and autoclave bags), biologic (spoke killing tests) or mechanical (check the thermometer and pressure gauge).

Chemical indicators of sterilization include color changing tape, color changing autoclave bags and various types of cards and kits. The simplest chemical indicator is a monochrome tape that verifies only temperature. More complex chemical indicators are typically multicolor and can verify the time, temperature and pressure of sterilization.

The more complex chemical indicator systems are referred to as "chemical emulators of sterilization" or "emulating indicator" or similar term since they claim to measure all the parameters of sterilization (time, temperature and pressure). Even so, this does not necessarily correlate with biological indicators. Only biological indicators measure killing of microorganisms.

In my lab each autoclave run has the monochrome tape type of chemical indicator applied and the results documented. This color change only takes place at very high temperatures and indicates the autoclave reached the correct temperature. It does not measure the time or pressure of sterilization.

Regardless of the type of chemical indicator you are using, the color change should be verified prior to disposal of the waste coming out of the autoclave. If the color change did NOT take place, something went wrong with the autoclaving, and the trash is assumed to be still infectious. The autoclave should be taken out of commission and not put back into service until the problem is corrected.

Below is a strip of autoclave tape that has NOT been autoclaved. This strip of tape is NOT showing the color change.

Below is a strip of autoclave tape that HAS BEEN autoclaved. This strip of tape is showing the appropriate color change.

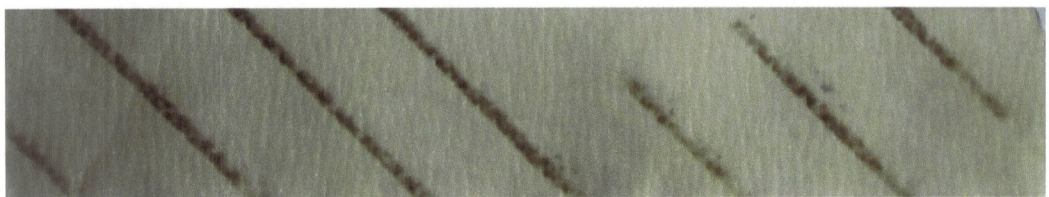

Biologic indicators typically contain spores from the most heat resistant microorganisms. Hence, killing all the spores confirms that your autoclave reached sufficient temperature and pressure for enough time to kill all the microorganisms inside the autoclave. However, if the biologic indicator shows growth, this indicates something went wrong with the autoclaving. The problem with biologic indicators is that the incubation takes hours to days such that results are slow to return. If your autoclave fails biologic indicators you won't know about it until the trash is long gone from your laboratory. You will then be trying to hunt down that trash to give it a proper autoclaving. If this happens, the autoclave should be taken out of commission and not put back into service until the problem is corrected.

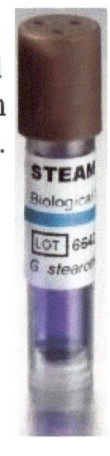

A biologic indicator typically comes from the manufacturer looking like this - a tube containing clear purple fluid. The tube is put in the autoclave along with a run of other items, autoclaved and then incubated. If the color stays the same and there is no turbidity this indicates NO growth of microorganisms in the tube. The test is a PASS meaning the autoclave worked properly.

The tube shown here is a FAIL - the color changed and the tube is showing turbidity. This indicates growth of microorganisms in the tube. If your biologic indicator is a fail, it means your autoclave did not meet the proper temperature and/or pressure for the required length of time. If you are not sure about a color change, compare the autoclaved tube to a new, unused tube. They should look exactly the same. Any color change at all is a FAIL.

Mechanical indicators measure the effectiveness of sterilization by directly measuring the heat and pressure using thermometers and pressure gauges. The autoclave in my lab prints out a piece of tape at the end of each run giving the pressure and temperature readings over the course of the sterilization cycle. After each autoclave run, the printout is checked to ensure the target temperature was reached for the minimum length of time. This printout is stored in a logbook to document the mechanical indicators of sterilization. If the autoclave did not reach the target temperature, or the target temperature was not held long enough, something went wrong with the autoclaving and the trash is assumed to be still infectious. The autoclave should be taken out of commission and not put back into service until the problem is corrected.

This type of printout tape is common on most modern day autoclaves. If your autoclave can't make printout, you could manually document the thermometer and pressure gauge readings over the course of the autoclave cycle. Here is an example of the autoclave printout tape from the autoclave at my lab, turned on its side to fit the page. This shows a successful autoclave run with the target temperature of 250°F held for 30 minutes:

```
AUTOCLAVE NO:1
LOAD NO:0013
OPERATOR: OK

D65  205°F  02P
D62  217°F  02P
E61  230°F  04P
E59  245°F  10P
S58  250°F  16P
S57  250°F  16P
S56  250°F  17P
S55  250°F  17P
S54  250°F  17P
S53  250°F  17P
S52  250°F  16P
S51  250°F  16P
S50  250°F  17P
S49  250°F  16P
S48  250°F  16P
S47  250°F  17P
S46  250°F  17P
S45  250°F  17P
S44  250°F  17P
S43  250°F  16P
S42  251°F  16P
S41  250°F  17P
S40  250°F  17P
S39  250°F  17P
S38  250°F  16P
S37  250°F  16P
S36  250°F  16P
S35  250°F  16P
S34  250°F  16P
S33  250°F  17P
S32  250°F  16P
S31  250°F  16P
S30  250°F  17P
S29  250°F  16P
S28  250°F  15P
H25  242°F  13P
H21  224°F  07P
H17  201°F  03P
H13  176°F  01P
H09  129°F  01P
H05  075°F  00P
H01  065°F  00P
MN   TEMP   PRES
DRY :05MIN
TIME:30MIN
TEMP:250°F
PROG:INS
TIME:23:09:03
DATE:01:11:18
Version:T04EAWP
```

Biologic indicators are considered preferable to chemical and mechanical indicators. Biologic indicators measure actual killing of organisms. In contrast chemical and mechanical indicators can only measure if the correct temperature and pressure have been reached for the correct length of time. However, biological indicators are more expensive, need to be incubated after the run ends and the results are not ready for hours to days after the autoclaving is finished. Chemical and mechanical indicators are more practical and inexpensive. My lab puts autoclave tape in every run and checks the color change immediately when the autoclave is opened after finishing. The autoclave printout is checked after each run.

Biologic indicators must be used in O.R. for every autoclave run where the instruments will be used for surgery. However, when autoclaving trash, you are not required to use biologic indicators for every run. When autoclaving trash, biologic indicators are typically only tested weekly, monthly, or after a specified number of runs or when changing the autoclave settings. My lab will test biologic indicators monthly or after 40 autoclave runs, whichever comes first.

If your autoclave fails indicators, check that the autoclave is not overloaded. If the trash bags completely fill the autoclave chamber they can block the flow of steam. Try autoclaving a smaller load and make sure the bags do not touch the walls of the autoclave chamber. Most autoclaves will keep an electronic record of their temperature during the run. Check this to make sure the autoclave reached the right temperature for the right length of time. If the autoclave did not reach the right temperature for the right length of time, take the autoclave out of service and call Maintenance or BioMed to fix it.

Some states and municipalities require permits to operate an autoclave for Regulated Medical Waste disposal. Before getting a new autoclave, check with your hospital's compliance office to see if any permits are required.

In general lab waste can be divided into the following categories. The disposal is different for each of these:

1. sharps including used glassware
2. solids
3. liquids

Does it go in 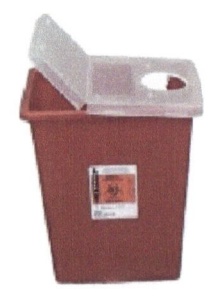 or 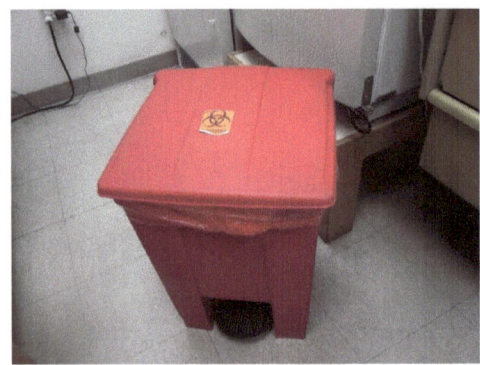 ???

Sharps go in the sharps container. Sharps are broadly defined as any object that is sharp enough to cut or penetrate human skin. This includes needles, lancets, scalpels, blades, glassware, etc. Glass slides and coverslips MUST be disposed in the sharps container even if they are not broken. Any sharp object can only be disposed in the sharps container even if it is unused (i.e. not contaminated).

Most hospital waste disposal policies state that intact glass tubes of blood can be put in the sharps container, but can also go in red bag trash if unbroken. Great care must be taken not to break glass tubes of blood when disposing them. In general, if you are not sure whether it goes in the red bag trash or the sharps container, put it in the sharps container. Better safe than sorry.

Sharps containers must be red, labeled with the biohazard sign, leak-proof and rigid walled (typically thick plastic or metal) so as to prevent punctures of the wall of the container. These containers must be easily accessible in any area where sharps are used. The reference is 29 CFR § 1910.1030.

These containers must be kept upright and are frequently secured in place to prevent spillage of the contents. Sharps containers are closed and discarded when they are only about three fourths full. There is a tenancy for the lab staff to overfill these containers. If these containers are overfilled they won't close properly and pose a risk to the staff removing them. As Lab Biosafety Officer you must be constantly vigilant to ensure that the sharps containers are being disposed before they overfill.

Non-sharp solid waste goes into either the red bag trash (contaminated) or white bag trash (not contaminated), except for chemicals which I will discuss below. Housekeeping will come as needed to collect lab's red bag trash, white bag trash, and sharps containers for disposal.

White bag trash (not contaminated) is the same as any other garbage. It can be disposed the same way as your household trash going into a garbage dumpster for disposal. The typical hospital uses white bags for uncontaminated trash such that the term "white bag trash" is persistent as a colloquial term for uncontaminated trash. However, the only regulatory requirement is that the bags can be any color other than red. Red is reserved for biohazard trash bags by regulation. If you look closely at the picture below, you will notice the trash can in my office has a yellow bag, not white. There is no requirement as to thickness, durability etc. and I have seen white trash bags so thin they tear easily.

The regulations governing contaminated trash state that this must go in trash bags that are red in color and/or have the biohazard symbol on it. Federal regulations require the bags used for contaminated trash to meet minimum tear resistance and impact resistance specifications. The reference is 49 CFR § 173.197. Some US states set higher requirements than mandated by the Federal government.

Red bag trash (contaminated trash) is considered Regulated Medical Waste (RMW). RMW is defined as waste that contains enough blood, body fluids or Other Potentially Infectious Materials (OPIM) to be potentially infectious. As a Lab BSO, you don't need to know much about the RMW regulations since housekeeping will collect it up for lab and dispose of it.

The regulations vary by state, but in most US states RMW can be autoclaved or incinerated and then disposed with other solid waste. Most hospitals I am familiar with autoclave their own RMW and dispose of it. Some hospitals hire an outside contractor to autoclave or incinerate the RMW and then dispose of it. In my experience outside contractors are not commonly used because they are expensive.

Does it go in 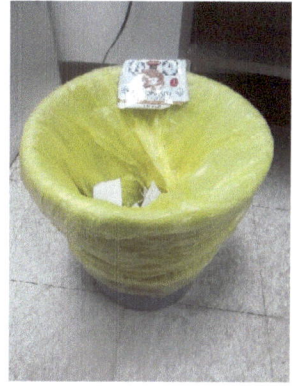 or 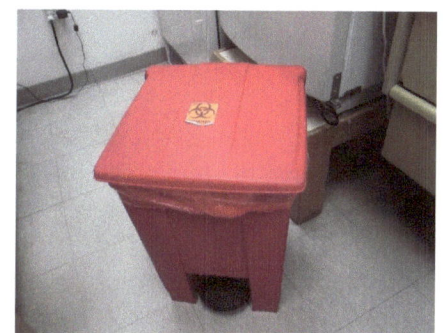 ???

As Lab BSO the most frequent question you will be asked is "Does it go in white bag trash or red bag trash?". The regulations require that anything visibly contaminated with blood must go in red bag trash. Anything that MIGHT be contaminated but does NOT have visible blood on it can go in white bag trash. In actual practice, if I am not sure which bag it goes in I will err on the side of putting it in red bag trash. Better safe than sorry.

For liquid waste, the main question is whether it can be flushed down the sink. It is acceptable to dispose body fluids (e.g. urine specimens for urinalysis testing) down the drain when done with the testing, provided that the patient is not known with infectious diseases that could be present in the specimen. For any potentially infectious fluid (e.g. pleural fluid for tuberculosis testing) autoclave the fluid first before pouring it down the drain. For certain chemicals, it is acceptable to pour small quantities down the sink with plenty of water. Consult your hospital-wide hazardous waste disposal office before pouring any chemicals down the sink. Any liquid chemical waste that can't be flushed down the sink should be given over to the hospital-wide hazardous waste disposal office for disposal. Solid chemical waste, such as powdered boric acid or sodium bicarbonate, follows the same pathway as described for liquid chemical waste – either flushed down the drain with plenty of water or handed over to the hospital-wide hazardous waste disposal office for disposal.

Chapter 14 – How to perform a laboratory risk assessment

The laboratory literature describes a multitude of different ways to perform a risk assessment. Some involve a list of questions with "Yes", "No" and "N/A" checkboxes. Others use elaborate spreadsheets with columns for risk, likelihood of an occurrence, likely severity, consequences of a bad outcome, etc.

There is no standardization. Multiple different organizations (APHL, CDC, etc.) have made their own risk assessment templates and recommend the use of their own templates as better than any other organization's templates. The various lab inspecting agencies (CAP, CMS, COLA, etc.) would be very unlikely to object to the template of your risk assessment, but could object if they felt the content was insufficient or incorrect. If your organization already has a risk assessment template you will likely have to use that template. If not you will have to devise your own template. In this situation, you could format your risk assessment any way you want and no one should be able to object.

A risk assessment consists of identifying the risks, estimating the likelihood of an adverse event occurring, and mitigating the risks. In the laboratory setting, this consists of evaluating the safety practices of your laboratory. This generally consists of reviewing lab safety best practices. Anything that does not meet best practices needs to be corrected. The general list of lab safety best practices is:

1. The facilities are adequate for all testing being done and the recommended containment levels are followed for all organisms handled. All lab staff have competency assessment for all procedures performed and equipment operated.
2. The lab staff always wash their hands after handling specimens and cultures, after removing gloves and before leaving the laboratory. Sinks are readily available in lab.
3. No eating, drinking, chewing gum, applying cosmetics, smoking, wearing jewelry, manipulating contact lenses, touching the face, no open-toed shoes or sandals, etc. are permitted in the work areas of the laboratory. Shoes made of water impermeable material (leather or synthetics) are preferred. Anyone with water permeable shoes (canvas) should wear impermeable, disposable shoe covers.
4. Any long hair should be tied back or covered by a cap.
5. Do not handle personal items (cellphones, smartphones, pocket calculators, etc.) while in the work areas of the laboratory. One of the most common contamination accidents involves a person in PPE whose cellphone rings. In this situation, people sometimes reach for their cellphone instinctively without thinking. It is best to have the lab staff turn off all their cellphones, smartphones, etc. before donnng PPE.
6. Food and drinks are not allowed in the refrigerators and freezers in lab's work areas. All refrigerates and freezers in lab's work areas have signage for "Specimens only. No food or drinks allowed inside". Check these refrigerators and freezers as to contents.
7. Safety goggles are required when handling infectious splashables.
8. No mouth pipetting is permitted.
9. The lab has a Biosafety Manual and standard operating procedures. The current versions of these are accessible in the place and at the time of testing. Check the Biosafety Manual and standard operating procedures to make sure they are present in lab, the information contained in them is accurate and represents current lab best practices, and all lab staff have acknowledged reading them and signed them.
10. The lab has policies for rejecting specimens received leaking or visibly contaminated.
11. Lab prohibits the smelling of culture plates to identify microorganisms.
12. All specimens, culture plates and stock cultures are properly labeled as to contents, date collected or prepared, etc.

13. All lab employees are familiar with the requirement to report accidents, injuries, spills, near misses, etc. Ask a few lab staff how and who a spill is reported to.
14. When an accident, incident or near miss occurs, the cause is identified and corrective action is taken to prevent recurrence.
15. All lab staff are familiar with the requirement to report work related infections and illnesses. Ask a few lab staff how and who they would report this to.
16. The lab has a disaster plan with Continuity Of Operations Plans (COOP). Check the lab's procedure manuals to make sure these are present.
17. Lab reports to Public Health all infectious organisms on the reportable disease list. This includes reporting of select agents (possible bioterrorism) to the CDC. Check the procedure manuals to confirm these procedures are in place.
18. The lab has at least two staff currently IATA certified to ship Category A high risk known infectious specimens. Ask to see their IATA certificates and check the expiration dates.
19. The laboratory has at least annual drills for fire, disaster, and public health emergencies (pandemic influenza, Ebola, etc.) as applicable to the testing in the lab. If problems are identified in these drills corrective action is taken.
20. Needles must not be recapped or otherwise manipulated by hand before disposal.
21. The lab has hard-walled, puncture-resistant sharps disposal containers and these are being properly used by the lab staff. Sharps are only discarded in the sharps container, not the red bag or white bag trash.
22. The sharps containers are not being allowed to overfill before disposal. Check all areas of lab for the presence of sharps disposal containers and check for overfilling.
23. Non-breakable items (plastic) are substituted for breakable items (glassware) whenever possible. Sharps with engineering controls (safety needles, safety scalpels, etc.) are used to the extent possible.
24. Broken glassware must not be handled directly. It should only be cleaned using a brush and dustpan.
25. Centrifugation and other manipulation of potentially infectious material capable of producing aerosols must be done under the BSC hood.
26. Work surfaces are decontaminated on at least a daily basis and after any spill of potentially infectious material. Lab's work surfaces are impermeable and easily cleaned. No rugs or carpets are allowed in lab.
27. Non-sharp potentially infectious solid waste is discarded in red biohazard bags. Observe several lab staff as they dispose of waste to see if this is being done properly..
28. Potentially infectious liquid waste must be autoclaved before disposal down the drain.
29. Materials to be decontaminated outside of the laboratory must be sealed in a leak-proof container before exiting the laboratory.
30. A sign with the biohazard symbol must be posted at the entrance to the laboratory and/or microbiology section. Other sections of lab have hazard signage as appropriate.
31. Laboratory personnel must receive appropriate training regarding the handling of infectious organisms, infection control, use of PPE, standard precautions and post exposure procedures.
32. Lab staff receive immunizations as appropriate to the infectious organisms they test for.
33. All laboratory personnel have regular health screening.
34. Access to laboratory is limited to authorized personnel only and is controlled by self-closing, locked doors. Check all entry and emergency exit doors to make sure they are working properly.
35. All persons entering the laboratory must be advised of the potential hazards and meet

requirements for entry.

36. Laboratory personnel demonstrate proficiency in laboratory safety practices before working with infectious agents.

37. Potentially infectious patient specimens are placed in sealed, leak proof containers before transport to laboratory.

38. Gloves must be removed and discarded after each use or after they become contaminated or compromised, whichever occurs first. The lab staff wash their hands after each glove removal.

39. Windows that open to the exterior must have screens. I would also recommend bars on the windows to prevent unauthorized access to lab.

40. Laboratory doors must be kept closed whenever work with biohazardous materials is conducted.

41. An autoclave is available in lab and used properly by the lab staff. Lab has all required permits for autoclaving and verifies the performance of the autoclave regularly using chemical and/or biological indicators of sterilization.

42. Any materials that must be transported off-site for decontamination are sealed in durable, leak-proof containers and packed in accordance with all regulations.

43. An emergency eyewash and emergency shower are available within 55 feet of the chemical hood and corrosives cabinet. Lab staff know the location of and have been trained on use of the emergency eyewash and emergency shower.

44. Access to cultures of organisms is controlled. The door to the Microbiology section is locked when not in use.

45. Biological safety cabinets are of the proper class for the work being done (typically Class I for BSL-1, Class II for BSL-2 and BSL-3 and Class III for BSL-4).

46. Biological safety cabinets have preventive maintenance at least annually and are certified for adequacy of air flow. Check the expiration date on the tag and check the most recent preventive maintenance and certification paperwork for the BSC.

47. Lab's BSC's are not located near airflow disruptions (fans, windows, walkways, etc.).

48. Lab staff are wearing appropriate PPE for the tasks being performed (gloves, lab coats, face shield, etc.). Check the lab staff's use of PPE in their routine work. Make sure they are donning the PPE prior to work with hazards and doffing the PPE when appropriate (no lab coats worn outside laboratory or in lab's breakroom),

49. PPE is readily available to the lab staff. Check the stockpile of gloves, gowns, face shields, etc. in lab's storeroom.

50. The lab has fire and/or corrosive cabinets. Check the cabinets as to contents and ensure there is no storage of incompatible chemicals (acids and bases, flammables and oxidizers, etc.) in the same cabinet.

51. Access to the fire and/or corrosive cabinets is controlled. The cabinets and/or cabinet room are locked when not in use.

52. The lab does not leave hazardous chemicals stored outside the fire and/or corrosive cabinets when not in use. Check lab's storeroom and work areas for hazardous chemicals.

53. Work with hazardous chemicals (pouring, mixing, etc.) is only done under a chemical fume hood while wearing appropriate PPE.

54. The lab staff have training on the proper handling, mixing, use, and storage of hazardous materials chemicals.

55. An SDS is present in the SDS binder for all toxic chemicals used in lab. Check that an SDS binder is present and check for completeness.

56. A formaldehyde exposure monitoring program is in place if the lab uses formalin.

57. Lab has fire extinguishers and spill kits. Check these as to expiration date on the tags. Make sure lab staff know the location and how to operate these.
58. Lab has emergency exits. All lab staff know the nearest emergency exit and the emergency evacuation plan.
59. All walkways are clear of obstructions, especially the walkways leading to emergency exits, emergency eyewashes, emergency showers, fire extinguishers, etc.
60. Thermal PPE are available for removing items from the autoclave and freezers operating below -20°C.
61. There are no obvious physical hazards in lab. Check for exposed electric wiring, wet floors, unsecured compressed gas cylinders, safe operation of equipment, ceiling tiles wet or discolored, etc.

When performing a laboratory risk assessment, you should have a checklist similar to the above. As mentioned previously, multiple different organizations make their biosafety checklists available on the internet. If your organization does not have a biosafety checklist you could borrow one from another institution. The above list is comprehensive enough that it could be used for most small hospital laboratory risk assessments.

The risk assessment is completed by going down the list marking each question as "yes", "no" or "not applicable". Any question that is answered as a "no" represents a deviation from laboratory best practices and needs to be remediated. If there are any findings during the risk assessment, the next step is to determine the likelihood and possible consequences of an adverse outcome, assign severity ratings to the findings then prioritize the findings.

The usual types of mitigation put into place in increasing order of effectiveness are: increased Personal Protective Equipment (PPE), administrative controls (signage, procedures, training, etc.), engineering controls designed to isolate the agent (physical barriers between lab employees and the agent), redesigning the lab, substitution (plastic bottles in place of glass, less hazardous chemicals in place of more hazardous chemicals, etc.) and elimination (removing the hazard from the workplace, such as discontinuing tuberculosis testing and sending all rule out tuberculosis specimens to a reference lab).

It is your responsibility as Lab BSO to ensure that remediations are put into place as quickly as possible for all findings. Give priority to any findings that could potentially have severe consequences. After putting remediations into place verify that all the risks have been addressed and the mitigations have been effective.

This is similar to how laboratory inspectors conduct their inspections with a set checklist of items to inspect. The only difference is that you will be inspecting your own laboratory. If you are part of a multi-site system, you will likely have to travel to all the laboratories in the system to perform a risk assessment on each laboratory. For all intents and purposes you will be acting as an inspector as you travel from site to site making risk assessments.

The risk assessment process outlined above should be done at least annually. It should be repeated if there are significant changes in personnel, equipment, procedures, methodology used for testing, after a lab move or renovation, before working with new biologic agent(s), after relevant new regulations are enacted, after a "near miss" or incident and/or with an increased level of security or threat.

When done with the risk assessment, the results are typically reported to the Lab Director, the Hospital CEO and any relevant hospital committees (Institutional Biosafety Committee, Quality Council, etc.).

This is typically informational unless the risk assessment has found significant problems that require input from the hospital's management. A copy of the risk assessment is kept in laboratory indefinitely.

Laboratory testing can be divided into three analytical phases. The preanalytic phase is everything that occurs before the testing – drawing the specimen, labeling the tube of blood, etc. The analytic phase is the testing. The postanalytic phase occurs after the test – reporting the correct patient's test results in a timely manner to the correct provider, disposing of the specimen, etc. The sum of all three phases is known as the Total Testing Process (TTP). The risk assessment should be set up to measure preanalytic, analytic, and postanalytic risks. The above list of questions covers all phases of the testing.

Chapter 15 – Shipping of hazardous materials to and from laboratories

Shipping of infectious materials is governed by multiple different regulatory agencies including the International Air Transport Association (IATA), US Department of Transportation (DOT), the Centers for Disease Control and Prevention (CDC), Federal Aviation Administration (FAA), the International Civil Aviation Organization (ICAO) and others. It is the sender's responsibility to ensure that the infectious material is correctly packaged and to follow all international, Federal, state and carrier rules and regulations. These rules and regulations tend to change frequently. Make sure you have the most recent version of each regulatory agency's shipping rules and regulations.

The penalties for a violation could be severe including substantial monetary fines, loss of your IATA certificate, your courier could refuse to accept further packages from you, etc. As the shipper of potentially infectious materials, it is imperative that you are familiar with and comply with all relevant rules and regulations.

Most laboratory specimens and supplies are shipped by air, so I will discuss the IATA rules first. IATA is a trade association of the world's airlines and sets international rules for air cargo. IATA has a classification system for dangerous goods. Known infectious substances are considered class 6.2 in this classification system. Class 6.2 is divided into:

1. Category A – high risk known infectious substances. These are given numbering as UN2814 for infectious substances affecting humans or UN2900 for infectious substances affecting animals (i.e. veterinary specimens) in transport.
2. Category B – low risk known infectious substances. These are given numbering as UN3733 in transport.

The packaging has to be very secure for a Category A high risk known infectious substance. The requirements are spelled out in IATA Packing Instruction PI620. PI620 specifies pressure testing, drop testing, puncture testing, water immersion testing, quality assurance, etc. for the packaging. You do not need to do all this testing yourself. All you have to do is to buy packaging from any vendor that sells packaging for Category A shipments with UN packaging markings indicating the package has passed the tests for Category A shipping. See the following pages for examples.

This involves multiple layers of packaging and absorbent materials to ensure that any spills or leaks are contained inside the packaging and do not seep out. Here is a diagram of the typical Category A packaging:

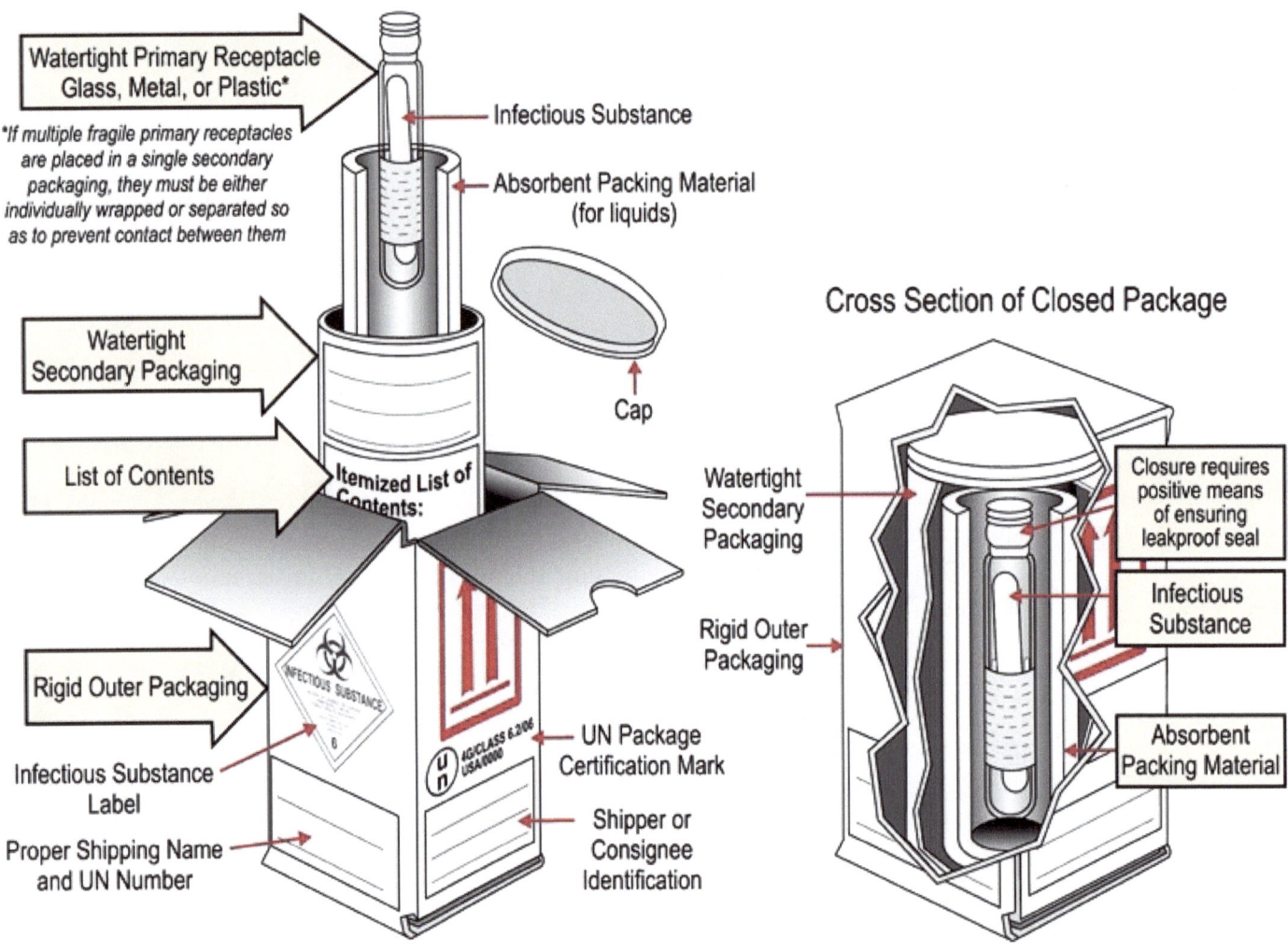

This type of nested, multilayered packaging is referred to as a triple packaging system. The three layers are:

1. Primary receptacle (i.e. the specimen tube of blood or container).The primary receptacle must be properly labeled, watertight and leakproof. It should be tightly secured such as a screw cap sealed with parafilm. If multiple primary receptacles are being shipped in the same box, they must be separated by cushioning to prevent breakage.
2. Secondary receptacle. A watertight, leak-proof receptacle to enclose and protect the primary receptacle. Several wrapped primary receptacles may be placed in one secondary receptacle. Sufficient absorbent material must be present in the secondary receptacle to contain any leaks.
3. Outer shipping package.

For Category A shipments the maximum shipping amount per shipment on a passenger flight is 50ml or 50 grams and on a cargo flight is 4 liters or 4 kilograms. The shipping box must have at least one surface with minimum dimensions of 100mm x 100mm. If you complete a shipping box and realize it does not meet the size requirement, you can put the completed shipping box in a larger box. This is referred to as "overpacking".

Required shipping labels and signs for Category A high risk known infectious shipments

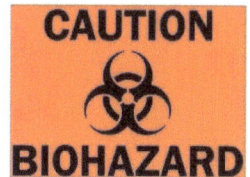

The biohazard sign must be present on all shipments of biological specimens. It must be fluorescent orange or orange-red with lettering and symbol in a contrasting color.

This end up sign is only applicable if the specimen is liquid.

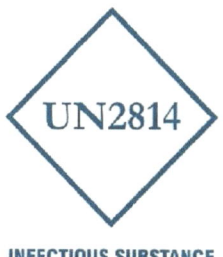

INFECTIOUS SUBSTANCE
CATEGORY A

The UN shipping number for Category A high risk known infectious substances affecting humans, UN2814, must be applied to all such shipments.

This sign is only applicable to Category A shipments that exceed 50ml or 50 grams. Such shipments are not allowed on passenger aircraft.

example:

4H"/Class 6.2/94
GB/2470

The packaging marking consists of:

➡ the United Nations packaging symbol
➡ type of packing
➡ the text "Class 6.2"
➡ the last two digits of the year of manufacture of the packaging
➡ State authority

These markings are UN packaging markings. They indicate the packaging is sturdy enough to meet the requirements in PI 620. This sturdy packaging is only required for Category A shipments.

All Category A shipments are required to be labeled with infectious substance signs.

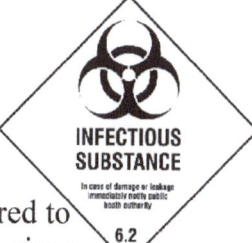

Every Category A high risk known infectious shipping box must have the name, address and phone number of the shipper and consignee (receiver) as well as the above appropriate signage. Category A shipments must also include the name and 24 hour emergency phone number of a responsible party on the shipping box. A requirement was added in 2018 that all labels and markings must be visible on one side, Here is what the shipping box looks like when you are done:

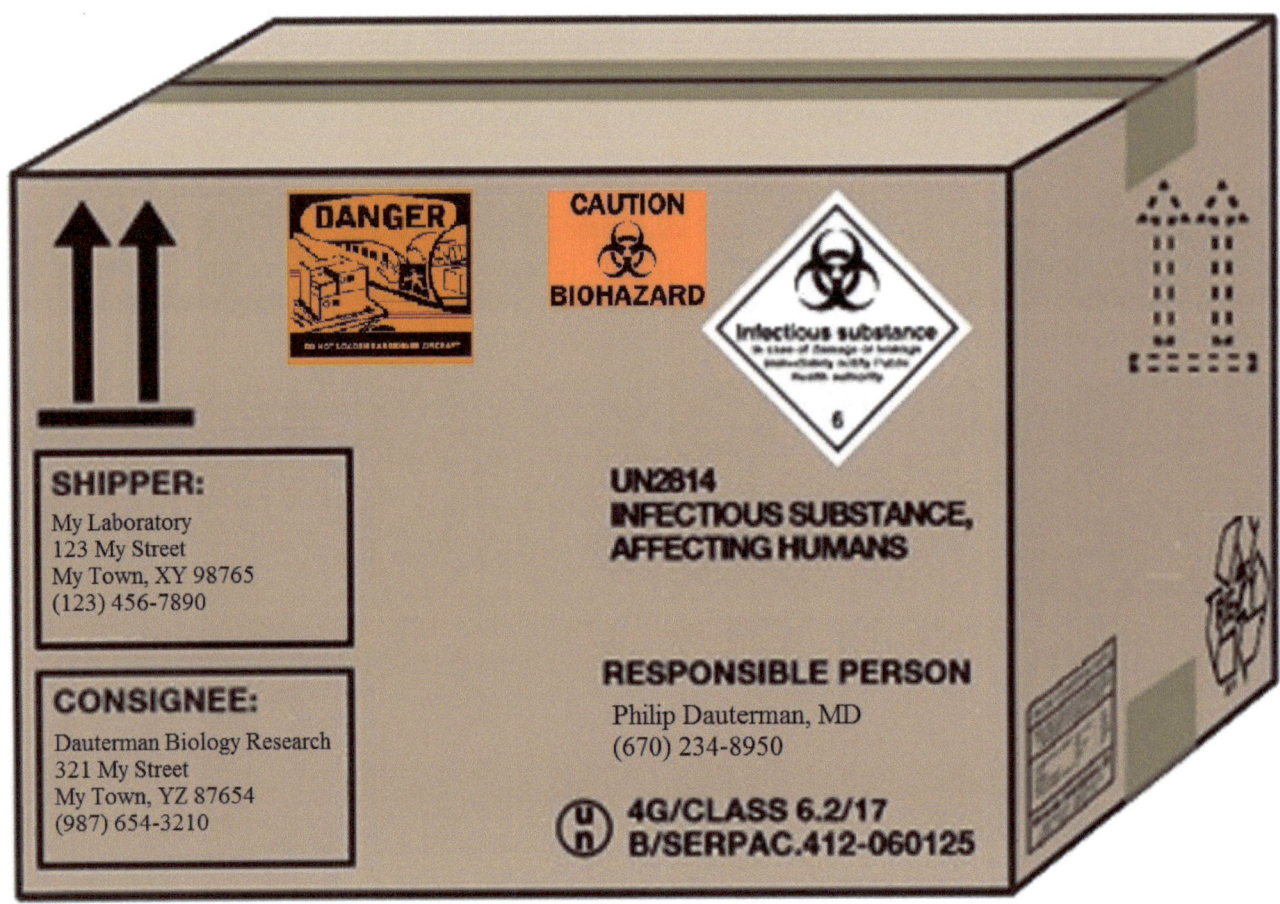

The required paperwork must be completely filled out with all information legible. The shipper will check this paperwork carefully before accepting the shipment and will not accept any shipment with incomplete and/or illegible paperwork. This paperwork is important because it contains the emergency contact information and other information that would be needed in case the box leaks. Category A shipments require the following paperwork:

1. Shipper's declaration form (completed by the shipper)
2. Air waybill
3. Import permit if the shipment is international (i.e. the sender and received are in different countries)
4. Itemized list of contents
5. Dispatch form and/or other required paperwork as needed

The requirements for packaging are less stringent for a Category B low risk known infectious substance. The requirements are spelled out in IATA Packing Instruction PI650. PI650 specifies drop testing, but does not require puncture testing, water immersion testing, etc. for the packaging. You do not need to do all this testing yourself. All you have to do is to buy packaging from any vendor that sells packaging for Category B shipments. Category B packaging does not need the UN packaging markings required for Category A packaging. Here is a diagram of the typical Category B packaging:

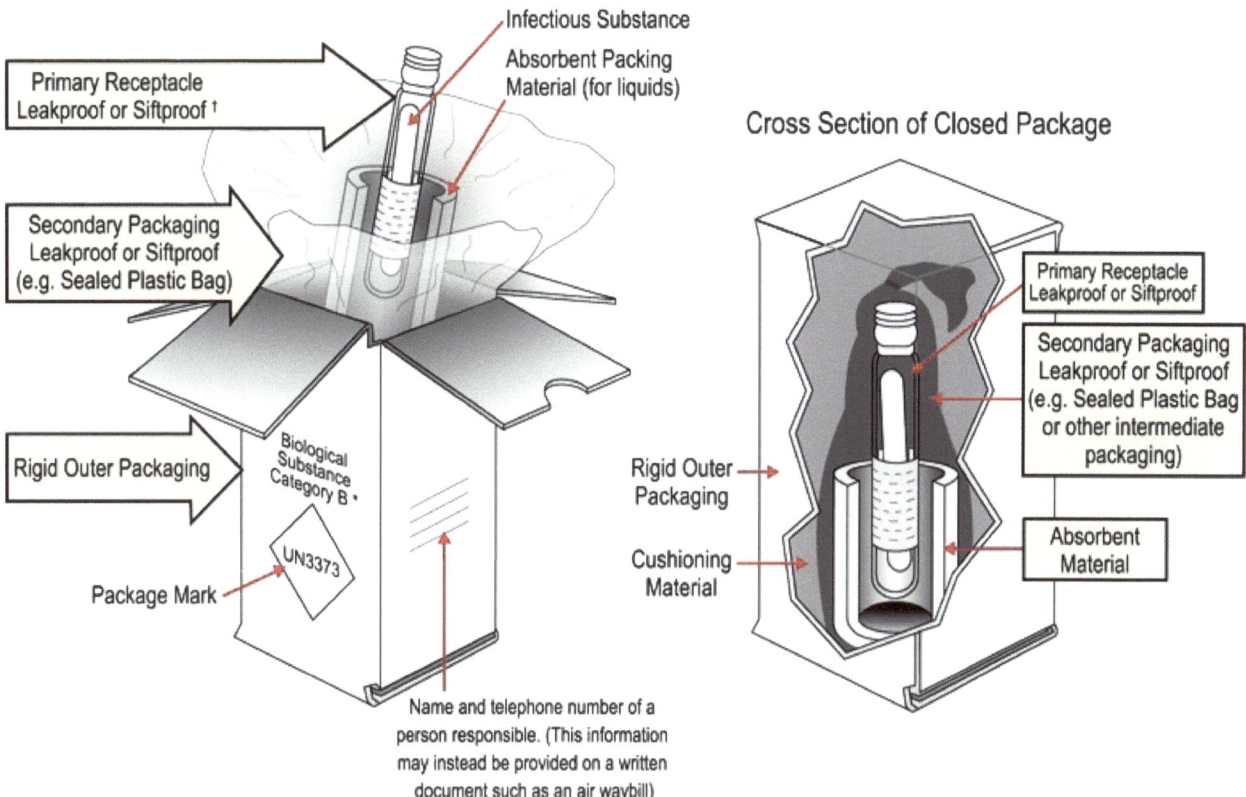

Notice that the Category B shipping container diagrammed above represents a triple packaging system of primary receptacle, secondary receptacle and outer shipping package. The maximum shipping amount per shipment is 4 liters or 4 kilograms. The shipping box must have at least one surface with minimum dimensions of 100mm x 100mm. If you complete a shipping box and realize it does not meet the size requirement, you can put the completed shipping box in a larger box. This is referred to as "overpacking".

The required paperwork must be completely filled out with all information legible. The shipper will check this paperwork carefully before accepting the shipment and will not accept any shipment with incomplete and/or illegible paperwork. This paperwork is important because it contains the emergency contact information and other information that would be needed in case the box leaks. Category B shipments require the following paperwork:

1. Air waybill
2. Import permit if the shipment is international (i.e. the sender and received are in different countries)
3. Itemized list of contents

Required shipping labels and signs for Category B low risk known infectious shipments

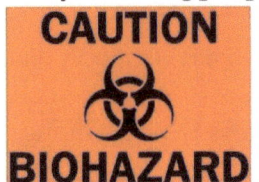

The biohazard sign must be present on all shipments of biological specimens. It must be fluorescent orange or orange-red with lettering and symbol in a contrasting color.

This end up sign is only applicable if the specimen is liquid.

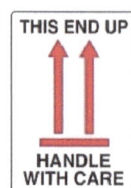

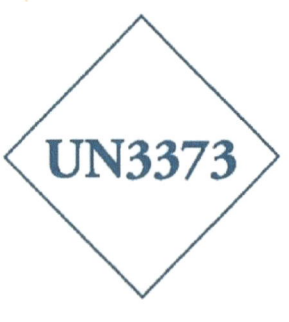

The UN shipping number for Category B low risk known infectious substances, UN3733, must be applied to all such shipments.

Every Category B low risk known infectious shipping box must have the name, address and phone number of the shipper and consignee (receiver) as well as the above appropriate signage. A requirement was added in 2018 that all labels and markings must be visible on one side, Here is what the shipping box looks like when you are done:

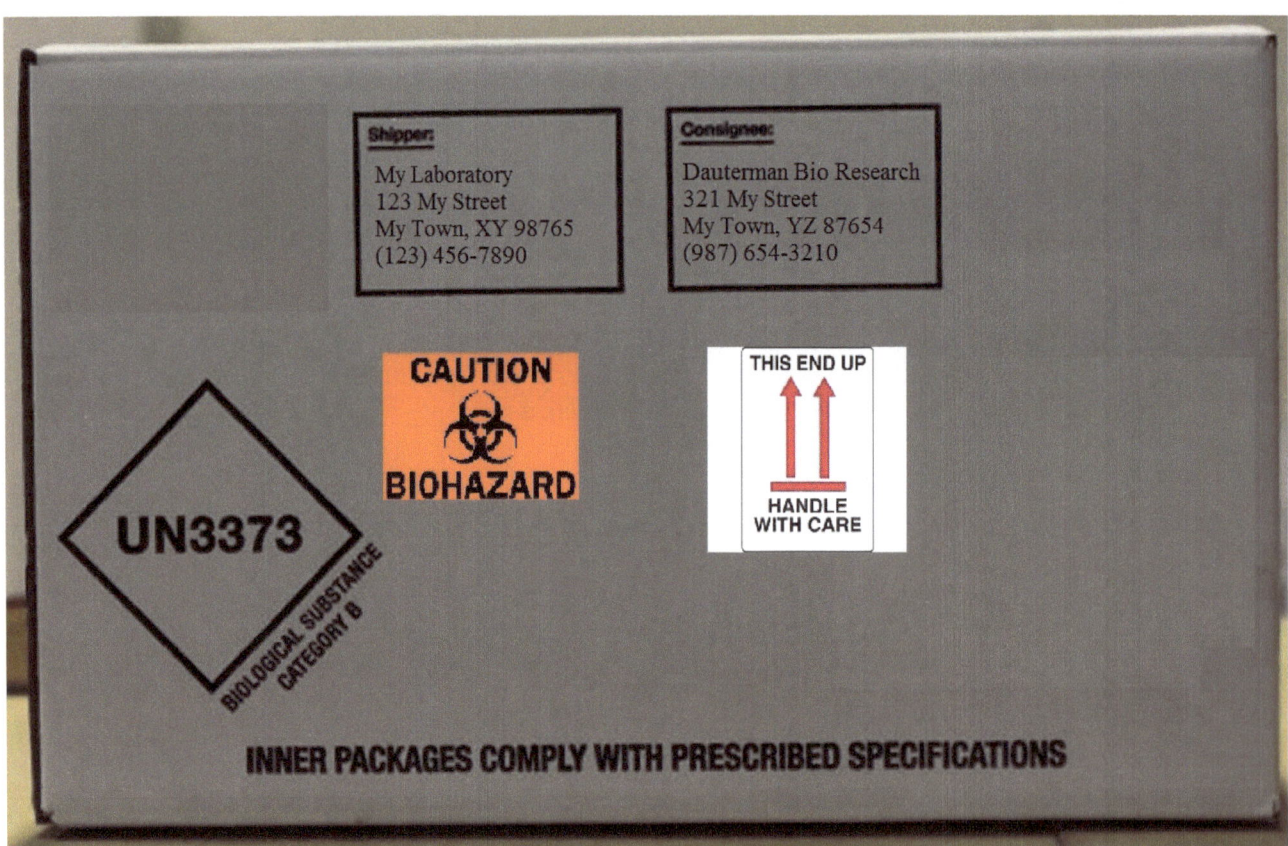

In comparison, a diagnostic specimen that is not known to be infectious requires much lass packaging. There is no regulatory limit on the amount that can be shipped in one shipment. This does not need to have any hazardous substance or dangerous goods markings on the shipping box. It can be marked as "diagnostic specimens, exempt, not restricted" or "human specimens, exempt" or similar. The typical packaging for a diagnostic specimen is:

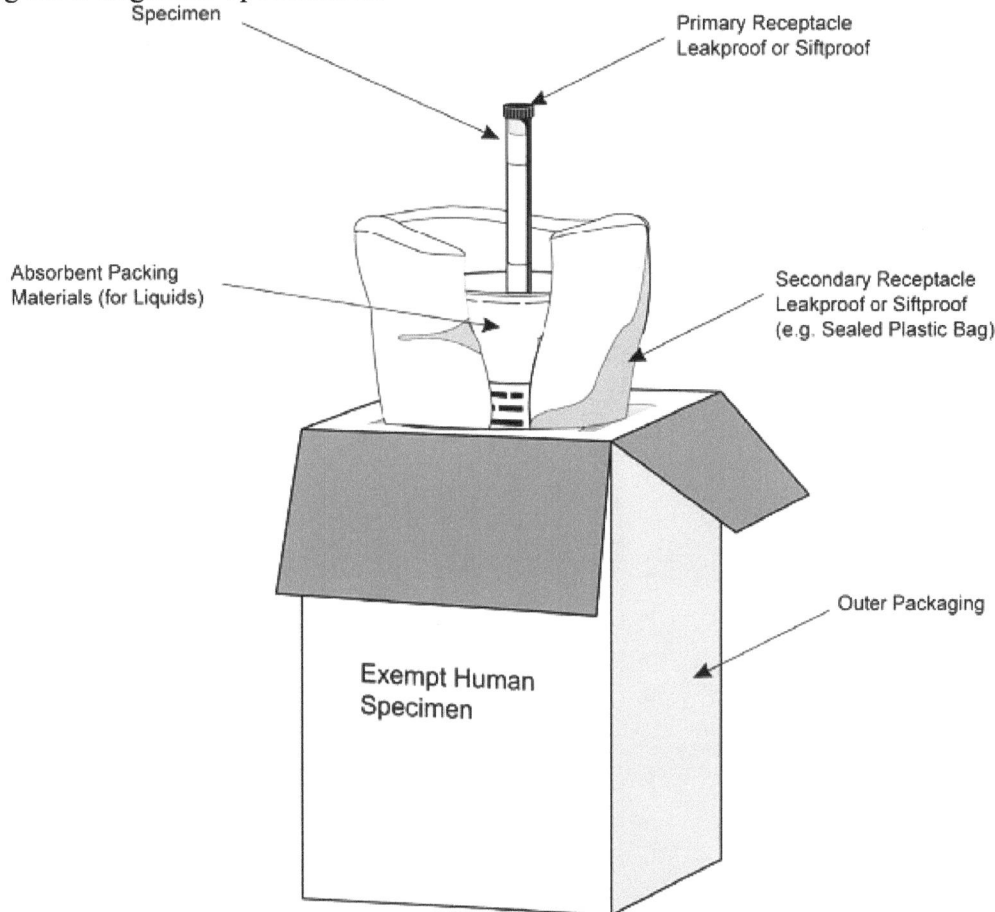

An exempt shipment of diagnostic specimens has a triple packaging system but it is less robust that the packaging for a known infectious specimen. The diagram above depicts only one tube of blood in the package. In my experience, shipments of diagnostic specimens to a reference lab typically involves 20 to 50 or more tubes of blood and containers of urine all bundled together into one box. There is no regulatory limit to how many specimens you can put in one box. You are only limited by the maximum container size and weight your shipper will accept. All specimen shipments must be packed with enough absorbent material to absorb ALL the specimens if the tubes or containers broke or leaked. This much absorbent material will be bulky and limit the space available in the shipping box.

The required paperwork must be completely filled out with all information legible. The shipper will check this paperwork carefully before accepting the shipment and will not accept any shipment with incomplete and/or illegible paperwork. This paperwork is important because it contains the emergency contact information and other information that would be needed in case the box leaks. For an exempt shipment of specimens the required paperwork is:

1. Air waybill
2. Import permit If the shipment is international (i.e. the sender and received are in different countries).

Required shipping labels and signs for exempt shipments

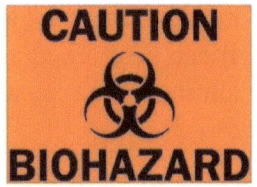 The biohazard sign must be present on all shipments of biological specimens. It must be fluorescent orange or orange-red with lettering and symbol in a contrasting color.

This end up sign is only applicable if the specimen is liquid.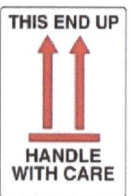

There is no regulatory requirement to have the sender's or receiver's name or address on the box; however, the shipper will likely require this the same as the shipper would require it of any other shipment. Here is what the shipping box looks like when you are done:

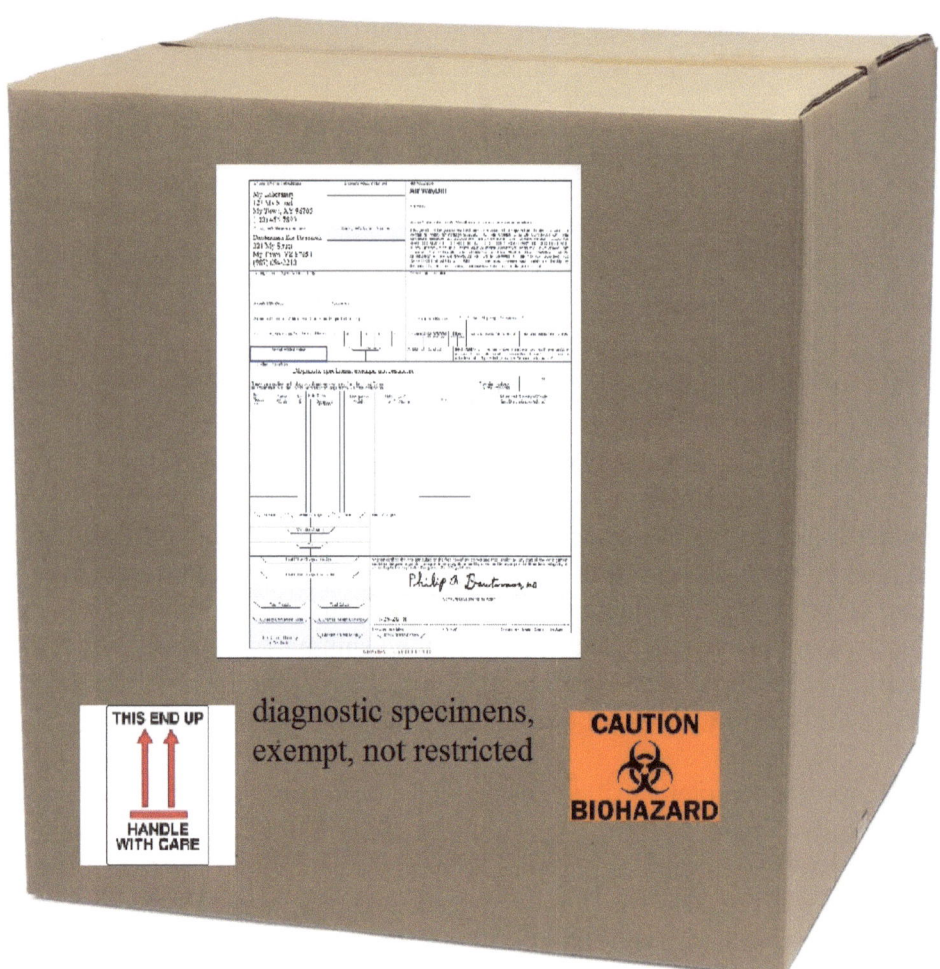

The air waybill is important, so I will give you a closer look at it here:

Shipper's Name and Address	Shipper's Account Number	Not Negotiable
My Laboratory 123 My Street My Town, XY 98765 (123) 456-7890		**Air WayBill** Issued by Copies 1, 2 and 3 of this Air Waybill are originals and have the same validity.

Consignee's Name and Address	Consignee's Account Number	
Dauterman Bio Research 321 My Street My Town, YZ 87654 (987) 654-3210		It is agreed that the goods described herein are accepted in apparent good order and condition (except as noted) for carriage SUBJECT TO THE CONDITIONS OF CONTRACT ON THE REVERSE HEREOF. ALL GOODS MAY BE CARRIED BY ANY OTHER MEANS INCLUDING ROAD OR ANY OTHER CARRIER UNLESS SPECIFIC CONTRARY INSTRUCTIONS ARE GIVEN HEREON BY THE SHIPPER, AND SHIPPER AGREES THAT THE SHIPMENT MAY BE CARRIED VIA INTERMEDIATE STOPPING PLACES WHICH THE CARRIER DEEMS APPROPRIATE. THE SHIPPER'S ATTENTION IS DRAWN TO THE NOTICE CONCERNING CARRIER'S LIMITATION OF LIABILITY. Shipper may increase such limitation of liability by declaring a higher value for carriage and paying a supplemental charge if required.

Issuing Carrier's Agent Name and City

Accounting Information

Agent's IATA Code   Account No.

Airport of Departure (Addr. of First Carrier) and Requested Routing

Reference Number   Optional Shipping Information

To	By First Carrier	Routing and Destination	to	by	to	by	Currency	CHGS Code	WT/VAL PPD COLL	Other PPD COLL	Declared Value for Carriage	Declared Value for Customs

Airport of Destination	Requested Flight/Date	Amount of Insurance	INSURANCE - If carrier offers insurance, and such insurance is requested in accordance with the conditions thereof, indicate amount to be insured in figures in box marked "Amount of Insurance".

Handling Information

Diagnostic specimens, exempt, not restricted

These commodities, technology or software were exported from the United States in accordance with the Export Administration Regulations. Ultimate destination   Diversion contrary to U.S. law prohibited.   SCI

No. of Pieces RCP	Gross Weight	kg lb	Rate Class / Commodity Item No.	Chargeable Weight	Rate / Charge	Total	Nature and Quantity of Goods (incl. Dimensions or Volume)

Prepaid	Weight Charge	Collect	Other Charges

Valuation Charge

Tax

Total Other Charges Due Agent

Shipper certifies that the particulars on the face hereof are correct and that **insofar as any part of the consignment contains dangerous goods, such part is properly described by name and is in proper condition for carriage by air** according to the applicable Dangerous Good Regulations.

Total Other Charge Due Carrier

Philip A. Dauterman, M.D.

Signature of Shipper or his Agent

Total Prepaid	Total Collect

Currency Conversion Rates	CC Charges in Dest. Currency

1/29/2018

Executed on (date)   at (place)   Signature of Issuing Carrier or its Agent

For Carriers Use only at Destination	Charges at Destination	Total Collect Charges

ORIGINAL 3 (FOR SHIPPER)

Below are the lists of Category A organisms current as of June, 2019. IATA maintains two lists, one for infectious substances affecting humans and the other for infectious substances affecting animals (i.e. veterinary). Any culture or specimen containing any of the following must be shipped as Category A. Any culture or specimen containing an infectious agent that is NOT on the following lists must be shipped as Category B. Any diagnostic specimen that is NOT known to be infectious is exempt.

Infectious substances affecting humans

Bacillus anthracis (cultures only)
Brucella abortus (cultures only)
Brucella melitensis (cultures only)
Brucella suis (cultures only)
Burkholderia mallei–Pseudomonas mallei–Glanders (cultures only)
Burkholderia pseudomallei–Pseudomonas pseudomallei (cultures only)
Chlamydia psittaci–avian strains (cultures only)
Clostridium botulinum (cultures only)
Coccidioides immitis (cultures only)
Coxiella burnetii (cultures only)
Crimean-Congo haemorrhagic fever virus
Dengue virus (cultures only)
Eastern equine encephalitis virus (cultures only)
Escherichia coli, verotoxigenic (cultures only)
Ebola virus
Flexal virus
Francisella tularensis (cultures only)
Guanarito virus
Hantaan virus
Hantavirus causing hemorrhagic fever with renal syndrome
Hendra virus
Hepatitis B virus (cultures only)
Herpes B virus (cultures only)
Human immunodeficiency virus (cultures only)
Highly pathogenic avian influenza virus (cultures only)
Japanese Encephalitis virus (cultures only)
Junin virus
Kyasanur Forest disease virus
Lassa virus
Machupo virus
Marburg virus
Monkeypox virus
Mycobacterium tuberculosis (cultures only)
Nipah virus
Omsk haemorrhagic fever virus
Poliovirus (cultures only)
Rabies virus (cultures only)
Rickettsia prowazekii (cultures only)
Rickettsia rickettsii (cultures only)
Rift Valley fever virus (cultures only)
Russian spring-summer encephalitis virus (cultures only)
Sabia virus
Shigella dysenteriae type 1 (cultures only)
Tick-borne encephalitis virus (cultures only)
Variola virus
Venezuelan equine encephalitis virus (cultures only)
West Nile virus (cultures only)
Yellow fever virus (cultures only)
Yersinia pestis (cultures only)

Infectious substances affecting animals

African swine fever virus (cultures only)
Avian paramyxovirus Type 1–Velogenic Newcastle disease virus (cultures only)
Classical swine fever virus (cultures only)
Foot and mouth disease virus (cultures only)
Goatpox virus (cultures only)
Lumpy skin disease virus (cultures only)
Mycoplasma mycoides–Contagious bovine pleuropneumonia (cultures only)
Peste des petits ruminants virus (cultures only)
Rinderpest virus (cultures only)
Sheep-pox virus (cultures only)
Swine vesicular disease virus (cultures only)
Vesicular stomatitis virus (cultures only)

The above list clearly delineates the specimens that are required to be shipped as Category A. However, the distinction between Category B and exempt shipments in not clear cut. The regulations state exempt specimens are "specimens for which there is minimal likelihood that pathogens are present". This is oftentimes a judgment call. For example diagnostic specimens being shipped to a reference lab for tuberculosis testing. The specimens are not currently known to contain tuberculosis, but there is enough suspicion to ship a diagnostic specimen. In this setting it is a judgment call to ship as Category B or exempt. If the clinical suspicion is low, I would ship these as exempt. If the clinical suspicion is high, the specimens will likely go as a Category B shipment.

Overpacking consists of putting the shipping box into a larger box. As discussed above overpacking is required for any Category A or Category B shipping box that does not meet minimum dimensions of having one surface at least 100mm x 100mm. Overpacking can be done for convenience so as to bundle boxes together. However overpacking needs to follow the rules discussed below.

All the inner packages must be properly packed, marked and labeled. The inner packages should not exceed the applicable shipping limits. The outer package must be labeled "overpack" and must be marked and labeled the same way as the inner packages. The outer package should be marked with the total amount of specimen in the shipment.

You are only allowed to overpack Category A shipments in the same box with other Category A shipments. Category B shipments can only be overpacked in the same box with other Category B shipments. You can't put Category A, Category B and/or exempt shipments together in the same overpack.

Here is a picture of an acceptable Category A overpack:

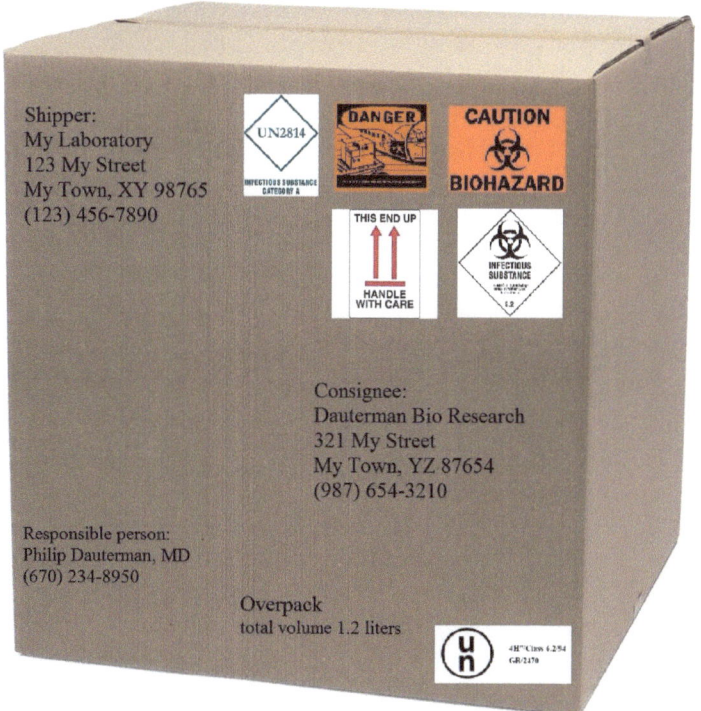

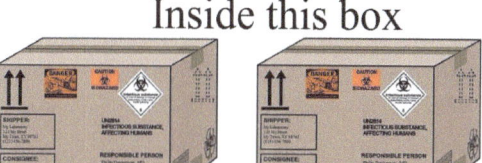

Inside this box

Properly marked and packaged Category A shipping boxes

Here is a picture of an acceptable Category B overpack:

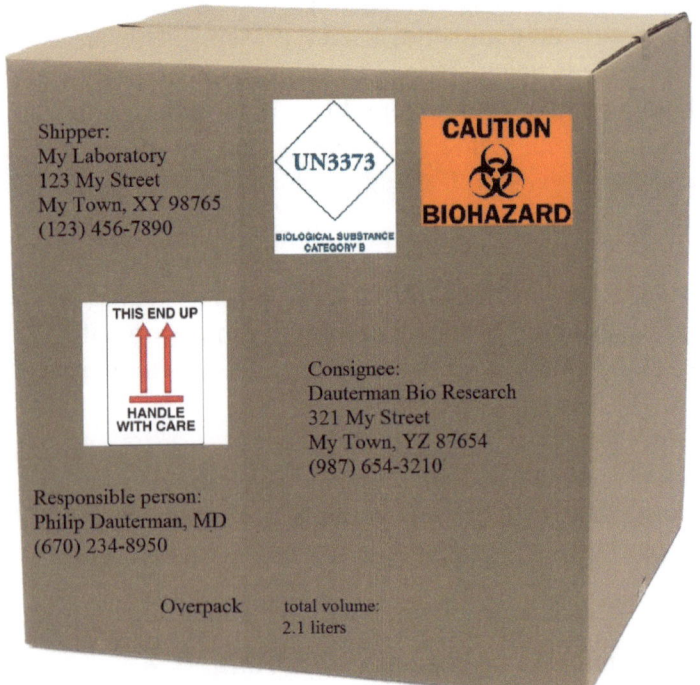

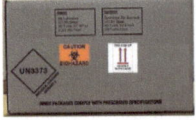 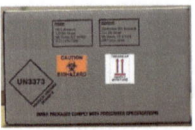 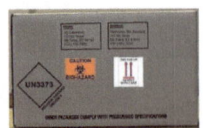

Inside this box

Properly marked and packaged Category B shipping boxes

When shipping frozen specimens, it is common to include dry ice in the shipping container. Dry ice is considered by IATA and the DOT to be a hazardous material in class 9 (miscellaneous hazardous substances). Dry ice is given numbering as UN1845 in transport. The IATA Packing Instruction for dry ice is PI954.

Any package with dry ice will need to have the appropriate signage on the front. For exempt and Category B shipments you will need to add a shipper's declaration form. For Category A shipments, add the dry ice information to the same shipper's declaration form that lists the infectious agents. You must write in the weight of the dry ice in kilograms on the shipping label. The limit per shipment is 200 kilograms of dry ice. My advice is for any package going long-distance or otherwise taking a long time in transit you should ask the shipper to re-ice the shipment in transit. Re-icing is more convenient and economical than sending a huge amount of dry ice with the specimens. Here is an example of dry ice signage:

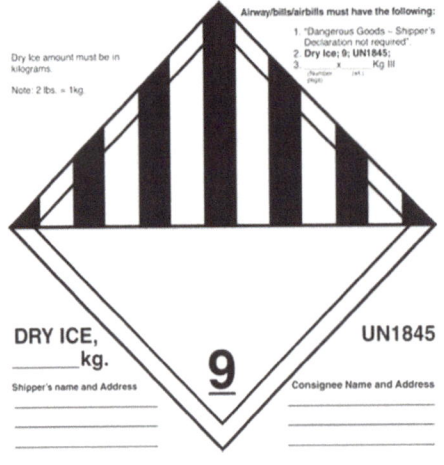

Training and certification in IATA shipping are required prior to packaging specimens into the boxes described above. The IATA training course for dangerous goods packaging is only 2 working days and the certification is good for 2 years before it expires. I have taken this course several times and it was a relatively easy "pass" each time I took it. However, I have been working in labs for over 28 years.

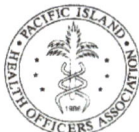

RECORD OF TRAINING

This is to certify that
Dr. Philip Dauterman

ON August 6th – 7th 2018 AT THE Royal Orchid Hotel, Tumon - Guam

HAS COMPLETED AND PASSED THE COURSE ON SHIPPING OF DANGEROUS GOODS WITH EMPHASIS ON CLASS 6.2 INFECTIOUS SUBSTANCES (CATEGORY A & B) AND RELATED HAZARDOUS MATERIALS.

THE TRAINING FOCUS WAS ON GENERAL AWARENESS, FUNCTION SPECIFC AND SECURITY AWARENESS FOR SHIPPING INFECTIOUS SUBSTANCES IN ACCORDANCE WITH THE 59th EDITION OF THE INTERNATIONAL AIR TRANSPORT ASSOCIATION (IATA) DANGEROUS GOODS REGULATIONS.

TRAINING PROVIDED BY

THE PACIFIC ISLANDS HEALTH OFFICERS ASSOCIATION (PIHOA)

THIS CERTIFICATION IS VALID FOR 2 YEARS FROM THE DATE OF TRAINING

Vasiti Uluiviti
M(ASCP)CM, MMSc, B.App.Sc., Cert (MLT)
PIHOA Regional Laboratory Coordinator/Trainer
Guam Public Health Laboratory
123 Chalan Kareta, Route 10
Mangilao, GU 96923
Phone: (671) 734-3338

Emi Chutaro, MSc
Executive Director
Pacific Islands Health Officers Association (PIHOA)
Pacific Guardian Center
737 Bishop Street, Suite 2075, Honolulu, Hawai`i 96813
Phone: (808) 537-3131

Always ensure the IATA shippers in your lab maintain current certification. My IATA certification given above was issued on August 7, 2018. This means it will expire on August 7, 2020. It is imperative to keep track of the certification expiration dates for the IATA shippers in your lab and ensure they renew before the expiration date.

If any IATA shipper at your lab has an expired certification he or she can't ship until the certification is renewed. If a shipper with an expired IATA certificate attempts to ship dangerous goods this could result in fines, criminal prosecution and/or other sanctions. This could be a serious problem for your laboratory. The IATA dangerous goods shipping course is available online. If any of your lab's IATA shippers have an expired certificate you should ask them to renew immediately using the online course.

When ground shipping biologic materials, the Department of Transportation (DOT) rules apply. These require similar packaging as for the IATA air shipping described above. For example the DOT requirements for Category A shipments spelled out in 49 CFR § 173.196 are identical to PI620, the DOT requirements for Category B shipments spelled out at 49 CFR § 173.199 are identical to PI650, etc. The DOT regulations are essentially identical to the IATA regulations such that proper IATA packaging will meet DOT requirements.

Shipping of hazardous materials chemicals is somewhat less stringent than the shipping of biological specimens described above. In all clinical laboratories I am familiar with, the lab will received small quantities of hazardous materials as reagents and supplies used for example to prepare stains (KOH prep, Acid Fast Stain, etc.) and will produce a small amount of hazardous materials waste. The waste disposal has been described in a prior chapter.

The DOT regulations are set up to regulate chemical manufacturers producing tons of chemicals at a time. For instance the DOT requirements to separate corrosives from other chemicals only apply to more than 1000 pounds of corrosives stored in the same place at the same time. The typical lab's shipment of one liter of hydrochloric acid to make acid fast stains is far below the threshold the DOT considers significant.

In terms of shipping, the packaging and shipping of HazMat chemicals falls on the vendor. All you have to do is receive the shipment, count up the contents, and move the contents into your fire or corrosive cabinets. The DOT puts quantity restrictions on the air and ground transport of hazardous materials chemicals. When lab is buying chemicals, it is the vendor's responsibility to ensure that all shipments of HazMat chemicals comply with all rules and regulations.

Only one time has a lab where I worked needed to ship HazMat reagents out of the lab. This instance occurred when a nearby lab ran out of essential reagents and asked to borrow some of ours. We had to figure out the shipping of the HazMat chemical on the fly, as we had never shipped out HazMat chemicals before, only HazMat waste.

There is one caveat here. Flammable chemicals, most corrosives and most compressed gasses cannot go on airplanes. They can only be shipped by ground transportation. If you live in a remote area, make sure you have a 3 month stockpile of reagent alcohols and acids for your acid-fast stain. From the time of ordering it could take months for the ground transportation of the alcohols and acids to arrive.

Another caveat is that all labs shipping dangerous goods are subject to inspection. The Federal Aviation Administration (FAA) is charged with investigating all complaints and incidents involving air shipment of dangerous goods. Make sure your shipping records are in order at all times. You could be inspected at any time and asked to produce your records. Inspections are not usually routine and usually only occur after some type of incident (e.g. an infectious specimen you shipped leaked in transit).

You as a shipper are responsible for ensuring all applicable transport regulations and requirements are met. This includes your responsibility to properly identify, classify, mark, label, pack, document and communicate information relating to all shipments you handle. Be careful not to overlook "hidden dangerous goods" such as pathology specimens being shipped in formalin containers. The formalin must be declared as a dangerous good, but this can be overlooked if one is not careful.

One final caveat is that handling the select agents (i.e. agents potentially usable for bioterrorism) requires security training specific to the select agents. Be aware of the current select agents list, and be aware that you cannot ship these agents, even if you have an IATA shipping certificate, unless you have the added security training.

Chapter 16 – Select agents and the Select Agent Program

The US government defines the biologic agents and toxins with the greatest risk of threat to public health as the "Biological Select Agents or Toxins (BSAT)" more commonly referred to as the select agents. The organisms on this list are determined by the CDC for human pathogens and by the U.S. Department of Agriculture (USDA) for animal and plant pathogens. Some select agents are on both lists. Below are the select agent lists current as of June, 2019:

HHS select agents and toxins (i.e. agents affecting humans)

Abrin
Bacillus cereus Biovar anthracis
Botulinum neurotoxins
Botulinum neurotoxin producing species of Clostridium
Conotoxins
Coxiella burnetii
Crimean-Congo hemorrhagic fever virus
Diacetoxyscirpenol
Eastern equine encephalitis virus
Ebola virus
Francisella tularensis
Lassa fever virus
Lujo virus
Marburg virus
Monkeypox virus
Reconstructed 1918 influenza virus
Ricin
Rickettsia prowazekii
SARS coronavirus
Saxitoxin

South American hemorrhagic fever viruses:
   * Chapare
   * Guanarito
   * Junin
   * Machupo
   * Sabia

Staphylococcal enterotoxins (subtypes A-E)
T-2 toxin
Tetrodotoxin
Tick-borne encephalitis virus
   * Far Eastern subtype
   * Siberian subtype

Kyasanur Forest disease virus
Omsk haemorrhagic fever virus
Variola major virus (Smallpox virus)
Variola minor virus (Alastrim)
Yersinia pestis

Overlap select agents and toxins (i.e. agents affecting both humans and animals)

Bacillus anthracis
Bacillus anthracis Pasteur strain
Brucella abortus
Brucella melitensis
Brucella suis
Burkholderia mallei

Burkholderia pseudomallei
Hendra virus
Nipah virus
Rift Valley fever virus
Venezuelan equine encephalitis virus

USDA select agents and toxins (i.e. agents affecting animals)

African horse sickness virus
African swine fever virus
Avian influenza virus
Classical swine fever virus
Foot-and-mouth disease virus

Mycoplasma capricolum
Mycoplasma mycoides
Newcastle disease virus
Peste des petits ruminants virus
Rinderpest virus

Goat pox virus	Sheep pox virus
Lumpy skin disease virus	Swine vesicular disease virus

USDA Plant Protection and Quarantine (PPQ) select agents and toxins

Peronosclerospora philippinensis (Peronosclerospora sacchari)	Sclerophthora rayssiae
Phoma glycinicola (formerly Pyrenochaeta glycines)	Synchytrium endobioticum
Ralstonia solanacearum	Xanthomonas oryzae
Rathayibacter toxicus	

Some of the select agents have further been designated as Tier 1 select agents, based on their higher risk of being deliberately misused with severe consequences to public health.

HHS Tier 1 select agents and toxins

Bacillus cereus Biovar anthracis	Marburg virus
Botulinum neurotoxins	Variola major virus (Smallpox virus)
Botulinum neurotoxin producing species of Clostridium	Variola minor virus (Alastrim)
Ebola virus	Yersinia pestis
Francisella tularensis	

Overlap Tier 1 select agents and toxins

Bacillus anthracis	Burkholderia pseudomallei
Burkholderia mallei	

USDA Tier 1 select agents and toxins

Foot-and-mouth disease virus	Rinderpest virus

The references for the above are 7 CFR Part 331, 9 CFR § 121.3 and 42 CFR § 73.3

The use, possession and transferring of select agents is regulated by the Select Agent Program (SAP). The CDC oversees the Select Agent Program. Any lab using or possessing these agents must apply for and receive registration from the SAP before handling or shipping these agents. Labs that are part of the SAP will have regular inspections by the CDC to ensure compliance with the requirements for handling and shipping of these agents. An SAP registered lab must have a biosafety plan, biosecurity plan, incident response plan, maintain an inventory of the select agents present on-site, have routine self-inspections, annual drills, etc.

The select agents are not the same as the IATA Category A list of organisms. For example flexal virus is on the IATA Category A list but not currently on the select agents list. SARS coronavirus is on the select agents list but not on the IATA Category A list.

The packaging used for IATA Category A is sufficient for the select agents. Some of the select agents are not on the IATA Category A list (for example SARS coronavirus), and in theory it would be possible to ship these in IATA Category B packaging. I have never heard of this being done, and the literature I have seen indicates all select agents must be shipped as IATA Category A.

Anyone handling the select agents must have special training, background checks, ongoing competency assessment, suitability assessment, occupational health screening, etc. These rules apply to the person packaging the shipment at your lab as well as any of the shipper's staff that will handle the shipment. These requirements will limit the number of shippers available to handle select agents shipments as typically very few shippers can meet these requirements.

I have spent my entire career working in labs not having SAP registration. Thus all my knowledge of the select agents and the SAP is second hand. This would be problematic if my lab ever identified a select agent. We would have no one qualified to ship the isolate out for further identification and workup. In this situation, the advice I have been given is if you are working up an isolate and you begin to suspect it is a select agent, you should discontinue all identification attempts immediately and ship the isolate out to a reference lab that is SAP registered. Thus, you will be shipping an isolate that is suspected but not known to be a select agent. At this stage of the game, you can still ship the isolate and it does not require select agent shipping. However, if you definitively identify the isolate as a select agent, the select agent shipping rules would apply and you would be unable to ship the isolate.

If your lab does not have SAP registration and definitively identifies a select agent, you would have to follow all select agent rules and regulations. Your lab would have seven calendar days to either transfer it off-site or destroy it on-site. You would be responsible for securing the select agent against theft, loss or release while it is present on-site. You would be responsible for filling out multiple forms including APHS/CDC form 4 - Report of the Identification of a Select Agent. Opening a Petri plate with the agent outside a BSC would be considered an accidental release of the agent. Anyone that has worked with the agent would need to have medical screening, etc. Given the extent of the regulation, it is best if your lab never definitively identifies a select agent. Thus, the recommendation to discontinue all identification efforts as soon as you first suspect a select agent and call the nearest SAP registered lab immediately to ask for help in dealing with the isolate.

The Laboratory Response Network (LRN) was established by the CDC for handling select agents, emerging infectious diseases, dealing with possible bioterrorism and other public health emergencies. These labs are all SAP registered. The laboratories I have worked in have not been SAP registered and in all cases the nearest SAP registered lab has been the State Department of Public Health Laboratory acting in its capacity as an LRN lab.

The Federal regulations governing the select agents provide severe penalties for violation. Thus, it is imperative to know the current list of select agents and to know that you cannot use, posses or ship these without prior registration in the Select Agent Program.

As a final caveat, the select agent rules and regulations only apply in the US. If you are outside the US and shipping these agents to another lab that is also outside the US, only the IATA rules and regulations apply, not the select agent rules and regulations.

Chapter 17 – Education and discipline of the lab staff on biosafety and biosafety related issues

Every job description I have seen for a Lab BSO lists workforce training and education. As far as I can tell from the literature this means Continuing Medical Education (CME) and not primary training on the basics of biosafety and biosecurity. Every lab tech had been educated on biosafety and biosecurity while in training. Thus, all lab techs should know the basics of biosafety and biosecurity before they start work. Their competency had been assessed before they began to perform testing independently. Their competency is assessed at least semiannually in the first year of employment and annually thereafter. Biosafety and biosecurity should be part of this competency assessment.

As Lab BSO, look over the documents used for competency assessment of the lab staff to ensure that biosafety and biosecurity are adequately assessed. If these are not being adequately assessed, ask the Lab Supervisor and/or Lab Director to add biosafety and biosecurity to the lab's competency assessment.

Many of the lab staff will be older and their training may not be up to date. They may need additional information on the latest emerging pathogens such as Ebola and Middle Eastern Respiratory Syndrome (MERS). Some types of PPE were not commonplace until recently, for example the full body suit with PAPR. These would all be good ideas for continuing education of the lab staff.

If you are working closely with the lab staff you should have a good idea of their strengths and weaknesses. Areas of weakness can also be identified by reviewing your most recent risk assessment of lab. If there are areas that need improvement concentrate on those areas with the continuing education. You can ask the lab staff what they think their needs are. In any event the CME should clearly communicate the expectations that lab staff will follow the biosafety and biosecurity rules and policies at all times.

Developing a CME activity is relatively easy. It typically takes me a few hours of internet research on any given topic to put together a 30 minute to 1 hour CME. Most CME are given as PowerPoint presentations. Make sure everyone in lab is aware of the time, date and place of the CME. After the presentation is over make sure to E-mail the lab staff with the PowerPoint presentation so they can review it whenever they want. In most situations when I was asked to make a CME there was no post test needed. If asked to make a post CME test, I typically put together a 10 question multiple choice test. The 10 questions deal with the most important topics of the CME.

The Lab BSO should be available to the lab staff during their daily work in case any questions come up. The list of potential questions is endless: How do we dispose of this particular waste? How does the new PPE work? etc.

The Lab BSO has the duties of enforcing the lab biosafety rules and regulations on the lab staff. The approach tends to be educational such as reminders to wash the hands when done testing specimens. If any staff repeatedly violates biosafety rules and regulations the staff involved should be written up. In this situation the approach becomes disciplinary as well as educational.

The Lab Supervisor should be present with you in any meeting that will be disciplinary towards any lab staff. The Lab Supervisor is responsible for carrying out any corrective (disciplinary) actions on the lab staff and should be involved, and probably also leading the way, for disciplinary action on any lab staff that repeatedly breaks the rules.

Chapter 18 – Lab Biosafety Officer leadership and communication skills

Most Lab Biosafety Officer position descriptions I have seen include leadership and communication skills. This is variously phrased as "able to work with stakeholders", "able to establish relationships with customers", "must maintain a working relationship with the lab staff", etc. These are phrased vaguely, and as far as I can tell relate to professionalism, leadership skills and other hard to measure qualities.

In my experience the most important aspect of leadership is your ability to relate to the people around you. A good leader is a team player and gets along with all co-workers. Try to be on friendly terms with all co-workers. The lab staff all have their own hopes and aspirations. Do your best to help them advance professionally (encourage continuing education and training). Encourage the personal development and career aspirations of the lab staff.

As a leader, a few basic qualities are necessary. A leader must be honest. If others can't trust you, they will not follow you. A leader should have a positive attitude, and lead by example. A leader should be confident, but should also know his or her limits. Always project a positive attitude, but don't "sugar coat" the situation by reporting things as being better than they really are. A leader should act in the best interest of the organization, be selfless and committed to the good of all. A good leader will be committed to excellence in the organization. A good leader is accountable and will admit to making mistakes. A good leader will never cover up his or her own mistakes and will not try to blame others.

A leader will plan and act proactively. Oftentimes, plans do not turn out as expected. A good leader will be able to rearrange plans on the fly based on the changing situation and will not act as if all plans are inflexible and unchanging. You should be able to handle unexpected situations. This may require creativity and intuition.

As a leader you must be able to communicate the organization's policies, decisions and changes to all employees you supervise. There should be open lines of communication and an open door to your office.

You as Lab BSO should be dependable, so as to earn the trust and confidence of those around you. As a leader, your goal is to contribute as much as you can to the organization by motivating the people who work with you. You should motivate the people you work with in a positive manner. Ask for the lab staff's input and opinions. Take seriously any suggestions for improving lab safety. Eat lunch with the lab staff on a regular basis and listen to their input. Don't say or do anything to another person that you wouldn't want said or done to you.

As a Lab Biosafety Officer leadership entails emphasizing the importance of attention to safety best practices. Recognize lab staff that show exemplary performance. Give awards for all goals met. Never berate or speak disrespectfully of anyone, even if they are not present at the time. Never criticize unless absolutely necessary. Even then, phrase it in a constructive manner. Be quick to thank the lab staff for a job well done. These practices will help foster a "culture of safety" where the lab staff have a feeling of shared responsibility for the lab's safety.

Communication can be defined as conveying information through written, verbal or nonverbal means either in person or remotely using technology. The information presented should be clear, concise and coherent. Communication comes in many forms – informational E-mail, signage on doors and fire cabinets, policies and procedures, attending hospital Infection Control meetings, phone calls to the epidemiologist and referral laboratory, verbal instructions to the lab staff, counseling for any lab staff that violates the safety rules, preparing and presenting Continuing Medical Education (CME) on lab safety, making oral reports to the Institutional Biosafety Committee (IBC), submitting written risk assessments to hospital management, etc. These all represent communication, and you as Lab Biosafety Officer should be able to communicate effectively in all these roles.

You as Lab Biosafety Officer should be familiar with your employer's rules for communication and sharing of information. Is it permissible to carbon copy informational E-mail to anyone outside the organization? I have seen people heavily criticized for seemingly innocent E-mail mistakes like clicking "reply all" and then discussing information that should not have been released outside the organization. Be very careful when you click "reply all" to delete any carbon copied E-mail addresses from outside the organization, and/or trim out any unneeded portions of a chain of E-mail before sending the reply. You as Lab Biosafety Officer are responsible for selecting the information you share.

Maintain professionalism in all communications. Keep a professional tone and demeanor at all times. Do not use vulgar language at work. Never become angry at co-workers or upset with them.

If you are giving a presentation, always try to stay on topic and do not digress. For any given topic try to have one or a few important messages to present. If someone asks a question that is unrelated to the topic of the presentation, tell them to meet with you immediately after the presentation is over to discuss their topic of interest. Then continue with the topic at hand.

I have not had much formal training in communication skills. The only formal training I have ever had in communication skills was a 5 day Association of Public Health Laboratories (APHL) Biosafety Leadership Workshop in September, 2017. I will summarize the contents of this course very briefly.

A news interview typically requires a great deal of preparation. The news organization will contact your lab or hospital and ask for the interview. Both sides must agree to the date, time, venue, topic of the interview, which topics are off limits, etc. If there is no agreement on these specifics the interview will not occur. You should prepare in advance of the interview by reviewing as much information as you can on the topic that will be discussed. You should have a general idea of the questions that are likely to be asked, and be prepared to answer them. It is helpful to have practice interviews in advance of the real interview.

When being interviewed there is a significant risk the reporter will have a political agenda and/or try to lead you astray. In this situation, the reporter will want to discuss topics unrelated to the intended topic of the interview. If this occurs, you should try to return the interview to the intended topic immediately.

The reporter may ask you to make "off the record" comments. In this setting, there is no such thing as "off the record". Everything you say could appear in the news media. Try to keep your answers short and to the point. If you have an important message to present, be prepared to summarize it as a "sound bite" of 10 seconds or less.

Do not provide any information that is not needed to answer the questions. Avoid using technical jargon or lab terminology that would not be understood outside of laboratory. If you do not know the answer to a question, state that you do not know. Do not lie, speculate or guess in an interview. Be polite in the interview. The reporter may ask questions intended to upset or anger you, but you should remain calm and friendly. Do not get into an argument with the reporter.

The interviewer may try to pressure you by asking questions rapid-fire. In this case, try to slow things down. It helps to repeat the question, as this will give you some time to think of an answer. Try to talk at a slow to moderate pace, even if the interviewer is speaking rapidly when asking questions.

Chapter 19 – How to write a policy and/or procedure

A policy is a statement of intent. It is usually dogmatic, broad and vague, stated in very general terms. For example: "The Lab will uphold quality patient testing". "The Lab will not tolerate unacceptable practices".

A procedure is a written document used to implement policy. It usually lists step by step instructions on how to do things, similar to a cookbook. For example: "add reagents and 2ml patient serum to the test tube. Mix gently then centrifuge at 1000 RPM for 5 minutes". Deviations from the lab's procedures can only occur under extreme circumstances, and usually require permission from the Lab Director or other authority.

A memorandum is a written document containing information usually of a temporary nature. For example: "Lab has run out of reagents for the CRP test. Please store all specimens for CRP testing in the refrigerator until the reagents arrive. The reagents are expected to arrive tomorrow". If a memorandum produces a permanent change, this change must be incorporated into the relevant policies and procedures.

The "procedures" in the typical lab procedure manual are really a mix of both policy and procedure. When I say "procedure" in this book, I am referring to the written documentation in the typical lab manual. Everyone refers to this as "procedure" even though it really is a mix of both policy and procedure.

The original copy of a lab procedure is referred to as the "controlled copy". Access to the controlled copy of the lab's procedures is strictly limited. Usually only the Lab Director, Lab Supervisor, Lab Secretary and possibly the section supervisors are allowed access to the controlled copy. You as Lab Biosafety Officer should be allowed access to the controlled copy of all procedures related to lab safety.

The controlled copy is usually stored electronically on the Lab Secretary's computer. When writing the lab's biosafety procedures you will be working closely with the Lab Secretary. All work you do on the procedures will typically be turned in to the Lab Secretary as handwritten changes, PDF files, Excel files, Word files, etc. The Lab Secretary will incorporate these into the controlled copy or replace the controlled copy with your new version.

There is usually a numbering system for the procedures with each procedure given a unique number. The Lab Secretary should maintain a master list of the procedures including the effective date of each procedure.

You as Lab Biosafety Officer should be aware of the chain of signatories for a new or changed procedure at your lab. Each new or changed lab biosafety procedure will begin the chain of signatories when you sign it as Lab Biosafety Officer. From there the procedure may or may not need to be signed by the Lab Supervisor and is always signed by the Lab Director. From there it may or may not need to route to other hospital officials – Director of Preparedness, Hospital CEO, etc. for signature. New procedures and changes to existing procedures are NOT effective until the chain of signatories is completed. In other words, you can't use a new or changed procedure until everyone that needs to sign it has already signed it.

Depending on your lab's inspecting agency, the Lab Director may need to review and sign all of lab's procedures once every 2 years. Be aware of the review requirements at your lab and ensure that the lab's biosafety procedures and manuals are signed for review in a timely manner.

Lab procedures are usually written in simple easy to understand language that tells the tech how to do the testing in a one step at a time, cookbook manner. The procedure has to be understood by the least intelligent tech in lab, so the language tends to be simple and clear. The procedure has to reflect what you are doing in real life and what you are doing in real life has to be documented in the procedure.

If your lab changes the way it does things, even a little, you have to change the procedure in the manual. The change is typically written into the hardcopy printout of the procedure present in the work area. It must be signed and dated by the Lab Director in order to be valid. These handwritten changes will typically be typed into the controlled copy of the procedure before your lab's next biennial inspection.

Most labs do not write the majority of their procedures on their own. They get their procedures from the test manufacturer or download the procedures from the internet. Another source for procedures is nearby hospital labs using the same equipment.

As a Lab Biosafety Officer, you will not be writing the majority of your own procedures, but you will need to review them all for accuracy. Things to check are:

1. Oversights and skipped steps are a common problem. Is the procedure complete? Does one step lead to the next, or is something missing in between?
2. Is it easy to understand? Is the least intelligent tech in lab going to have a hard time reading and understanding it?
3. Could a lab tech new to this workplace read the procedure, and do the test without supervision and without asking for help?
4. Does the written procedure reflect what is being done in real life? If a specific manufacturer is named, are we still using that manufacturer?
5. Does it accurately convey the manufacturer's instructions and lab best practices?
6. Has anything changed since the time the procedure was written?

For each procedure, the date of creation and each date of modification is typed into the procedure. After a procedure is no longer needed, it is retired to the retired procedure folder. The retirement date is logged in the retired procedure logbook. Retired procedures should be kept at least two years before disposal.

I will give an example of a procedure on the next three pages. This is the lab-wide Biohazard Waste Disposal procedure.

MY LAB
LAB GENERAL PROCEDURE MANUAL

CATEGORY: **OPERATIONS/MANAGEMENT**	**CODE: 3145**
SUBJECT: **Biohazard Waste Disposal**	**EFFECTIVE: 1/14/2019**
RESPONSIBLE DEPARTMENT/DESIGNEE: **Laboratory**	**PAGE: 1 of 3**

PURPOSE:

To provide guidelines for the handling and disposal of Biohazard waste.

DEFINITION:

• Clinical laboratory biohazardous waste includes cultures of etiologic agents, equipment, instruments, sharps, dressing and other disposable materials, which when used and contaminated are likely to contain infectious agents.

• Clinical laboratory specimens include tissues, blood, excreta and secretions. These potentially contain infectious agents.

• Other Potentially Infectious Material (OPIM) includes any bodily fluid not listed above and any other material which presents a significant risk of infection because it is contaminated with, or may reasonably be expected to be contaminated with, infectious agents.

• Non-infectious waste includes any waste products NOT visibly contaminated with blood and never in contact with contaminated bodily fluids or cultures. These should NOT be placed in the red bags used for biohazardous waste. Instead these items go in white bag trash.

POLICY:

• All requirements set forth by this policy on Biohazardous Waste shall be followed as outlined and shall be applied to all biohazardous waste generated.

• Infectious sharps shall be contained for disposal in leak-proof, rigid and puncture resistant containers, such as plastic or metal. When three quarters filled close the lid securely to preclude loss of the contents prior to discarding.

• Cultures of viable etiologic agents shall be rendered noninfectious before disposal by heating in a steam autoclave or by another sterilization technique approved in writing by the facility.

- Standard Precautions are utilized during the handling of all biohazardous wastes.

- Biohazardous waste shall be kept separated from non-biohazardous waste at the point of origin.

- Containers used for biohazardous waste shall be kept secured in locked areas so as to deny access to unauthorized persons.

- Biohazardous waste shall not be stored for more than one (1) day, other than sharps disposal containers.

- All biohazardous waste, except sharps, will be single-bagged prior to disposal.

- The following items are considered biohazardous and disposed of according to this procedure:

    1. Used needles, syringes and glassware
    2. Lab specimens including blood, tissue, urine, feces, and bodily fluids
    3. Used disposable surgical blades and all other contaminated sharps
    4. Used culture plates
    5. Used culture swabs
    6. Any materials in contact with either blood or bloody drainage
    7. Any disposable item in direct contact with a wound or person with a communicable disease

- Dispose of all biohazardous wastes appropriately in sharps containers or in red plastic bags located in designated covered waste containers with foot pedals.

PROCEDURE:

- Used culture plates are to be collected in red autoclavable biohazard bags and autoclaved for disposal.

- Urine specimens can be poured down the sink or toilet followed by large amounts of water. Empty urine containers are thrown into red bag biohazard trash.

- Stool specimens are to be flushed down the toilet. Empty stool containers are thrown into red bag biohazard trash.

- Used needles, syringes, lancets, scalpels and all other contaminated sharps are disposed of in the hard plastic or metal sharps disposal containers.

- Never recap a needle. Never reach inside the sharps disposal container. Close the lid securely on every three quarters filled sharps disposal container, prior to discarding. Never dispose of syringes or needles in a general trash receptacle.

- Used tubes of blood can be disposed in red bag trash or in sharps containers. Be careful not to break the tubes when dropping them in the red bag trash or the sharps containers.

- When each red bag fills and/or at the end of each day, follow the bagging procedure.

    1. Remove the bag and contents from the red trash container and close the container securely.

    2. Unfold cuff and tie it closed securely, being careful not to touch the inside of the bag.

    3. Place the red bag next to a trash container to be picked up by Environmental Services personnel.

    4. Carefully pick up a new clean red bag. Check the new bag for integrity (no holes in the new bag). Line the trash container with it.

    5. Remove your gloves and throw them in a contaminated trash container.

    6. Wash your hands.

    7. Call Environmental Services for immediate disposal of the full red bag.

REVIEWED AND APPROVED BY:

Philip A. Dauterman, M.D.

_____   _1/14/2019_____
Laboratory Biosafety Officer   Date

_____   _____
Lab Supervisor   Date

Philip A. Dauterman, M.D.

_____   _1/14/2019_____
Lab Director   Date

**Reviewed Last
(Date and Initial)**

_____

_____

_____

Chapter 20 – How to write a lab Biosafety Manual

The Lab Biosafety Officer is charged with making the Biosafety Manual. The Biosafety Manual is a collection of all the policies and procedures that relate to safety in the lab. The prior chapter dealt with making an individual policy and/or procedure. When making a Biosafety Manual you need to make a policy and/or procedure for each aspect of lab safety and then collect all these policies and procedures into a single binder with appropriate numbering, table of contents, etc.

This is not as difficult as it sounds. The principles of biosafety are universal at all labs. Therefore you can largely copy and paste any biosafety manual from any other organization with the same equipment and biosafety containment level you have.

I will put my lab's Biosafety Manual on the following pages, edited to remove the names. My lab is a BSL-2 lab. If your lab uses BSL-2 you could largely copy and paste this and use it as your own Biosafety Manual. If your lab is using BSL-2+, BSL-3 or BSL-4 you could use a Biosafety Manual from a similar lab as your template.

MY LABORATORY   BIOSAFETY MANUAL

Table of Contents

MY LABORATORY   BIOSAFETY MANUAL

PURPOSE

This manual applies to all staff, visitors, guests, volunteers, building staff, contractors, service staff and all others who enter the laboratory. The Lab Director will review this manual biennially for changes or corrections to ensure that it is accurate.

BACKGROUND

I. Introduction to General Safety and Training for the BSL-2 Laboratory

A. Required Training

1. The minimum qualification to work in a BSL-2 lab are:
   a) Training including Biosafety, Lab Safety, Infection Control, HIPAA, Fire Safety and Fire Prevention (also Radiation Safety if applicable).
   b) Certified Laboratory technician, technologist or phlebotomist.

2. Laboratory personnel shall demonstrate the following:
   a) Willingness to follow established laboratory safety guidelines and standard operating procedures.
   b) Proficiency in donning and doffing PPE.
   c) Proficiency in handling potentially infectious specimens.

3. This document will provide the basis of training.

The Lab Director & Lab BSO will provide information and arrange for training at the time of an individual's initial assignment to the lab and will arrange refresher trainings annually and when there are any changes in processes or procedures.

B. Administrative Procedures

It is the responsibility of each employee to consider carefully every action taken in the BSL-2 lab and its potential impact on possible exposure or contamination, and to follow established Standard Operating Procedures (SOPs) and protocols diligently and without variance.

1. All employees will read and adhere to the Biosafety Manual and to the SOP Manual. All employees will use pertinent sections in the Biosafety in Microbiological and Biomedical Laboratories, CDC-NIH, 5th edition as a guideline and reference.

2. All employees working in the lab will be offered Hepatitis B vaccine and other vaccines as applicable to the testing they perform.

3.   No employee will be trained to work in the lab without the express permission of the Lab Director and Lab BSO.

4.   New or changed SOPs and protocols must be approved by the Lab Director before use. New or changed SOPs and protocols involving biosafety additionally need the approval of the Lab BSO.

5.   Current SOPs and protocols will be reviewed and/or revised by the Laboratory Director every 2 years.

C. Description of Laboratory

The Laboratory is located in the Hospital Building on the second floor in the main hallway. Floor diagrams are displayed as Appendix A at the end of this manual. The locations of the sinks, emergency eyewashes and showers, fire extinguisher, fire blanket, fuse box, exits, and telephones are included in the diagram.

D. General Laboratory Safety

Work with infectious agents is performed in the Microbiology Lab.

1.   Laboratory employees must immediately notify the laboratory supervisor or laboratory director in case of an accident, injury, illness, or overt exposure associated with laboratory activities.

2.   No eating, drinking, smoking including e-cigarette, chewing of betel nut, handling contact lenses, or applying cosmetics is permitted in the lab at any time.

3.   No animals or minors (persons under the age of 18), or immunocompromised persons will be allowed to enter the lab at any time.

4.   Food, medications, or cosmetics should not be brought into the lab for storage or later use. Food is stored outside in areas designated specifically for that purpose.

5.   No open-toed shoes or sandals are allowed in the laboratory.

6.   PPE including gloves, lab coat, and eye protection should be worn as needed.

7.   All skin defects such as cuts, abrasions, ulcers, areas of dermatitis, etc. should be covered with an occlusive bandage.

8.   Mouth pipetting is prohibited; mechanical pipetting devices are to be used at all times.

9. All procedures are to be performed carefully to minimize the creation of splashes or aerosols.

10. Follow all manufacturer's instructions and SOPs when using any of the laboratory equipment.

11. Wash hands:
    a) after removing gloves, and
    b) before leaving the laboratory.

12. Razor blades, scalpels, and hypodermic needles ("sharps") should be discarded into sharps disposal containers. DO NOT recap needles.

13. Work surfaces will be decontaminated daily and as needed with bleach or other approved disinfectant. Follow manufacturer instructions for contact time.

14. All cultures, stocks, and other regulated wastes are decontaminated by autoclaving before disposal.

E. General Biosafety Cabinet Safety

1. Wash your hands and don the appropriate PPE. Gloves and lab coat must be worn at all times. Raise the window sash on the cabinet to the appropriate height. Turn on the BSC's fans at least 10 minutes before placing infectious materials into the cabinet.

2. Load the cabinet with the necessary cultures, reagents and supplies. Keep the clean items at least 12 inches separated from the contaminated items. Place a red bag trash container inside the cabinet. If working with sharps, place a sharps disposal container in the BSC.

3. Check the certification sticker and Magnehelic Gauge to verify that the biosafety cabinet is working properly. Do NOT use the biosafety cabinet if the air flow is not in range. If the air flow is out of range report this to the Lab BSO and/or Lab Director immediately.

4. While working, DO NOT disrupt the airflow through the hood by placing ANY item on the grilles or by opening the door to the corridor. Work from the clean to the dirty areas of the cabinet.

5. In general, the interior of the BSC should be considered to be a contaminated zone, even though every effort is made to keep the surfaces clean. Dispose all waste from the BSC in the red trash bag or sharps disposal container as appropriate. Dispose of these properly after finishing.

6.   After use, disinfect anything that has been inside the cabinet (media bottles, etc.) before taking it out. Clean the interior surfaces of the BSC with 10% bleach after completion of work. Follow with 70% alcohol. Allow the BSC's fans to run for at least 10 minutes following use. Make sure the BSC's fans are off before leaving.

F. General Accident Procedures

1.   Spills - Open the Biosafety Spill Kit and drop the disinfectant absorbent pads onto the spill. If no spill kit is available, apply paper towels to absorb the spill, and then soak paper towels with 10% bleach. For spills outside the biosafety cabinet, alert others in the area. Use N95 respirator mask if there is a possibility of harmful aerosols.

2.   Follow all aspects of the emergency SOPs without exception.

II. Standard Operating Procedures

A. 1000 – Containment Requirements

1001 – Laboratory Entry/Exit

1001.1 Entering the lab to begin work

     a) Put on personal protective equipment including gloves and gown or lab coat.

     b) Gather all materials for the testing.

1001.2 Exiting Laboratory

Before exiting the lab, be sure that all required documentation has been completed, the hood and work area are clean, all contaminated waste materials are disposed of properly, and stocks have been returned to the proper storage area. Wash your hands.

1002 - Specimen Transport

Transport of biological materials to another building or lab within the same building should be done in a covered, sealed container. If the samples are infectious, use a secondary container and label it with the contents and a contact person/phone number.

1003 - Work within the Laboratory

1003.1 The user should verify inward airflow of the biological safety cabinet before initiating work by checking the Magnehelic Gauge.

1003.2 All work should be done within the operationally effective zone of the biological safety cabinet.

1003.3 Discard pipettes and tips appropriately in red biohazard bins.

1003.4 The interior of the hood should be cleaned periodically.

1003.5 When vacuum lines are used with systems containing agents, they will be protected with in-line filters to prevent entry of agents into the lines, and will be protected by a liquid trap containing bleach. No liquid should be allowed into any drain connected to the sanitary sewer system (e.g. from a sink) unless first autoclaved.

B. 2000 – Proper Use and Maintenance of Equipment

2001 - Biological Safety Cabinets

2001.1 – To assure containment of aerosols inside the cabinet and establish proper air flow for containment, the BSC's fans should be turned on at least ten minutes before infectious materials are to be put into the biosafety cabinet.

2001.2 – Biosafety cabinets must be certified by a qualified outside contractor prior to use and annually thereafter. Check the certification sticker on the front of the unit to verify your biosafety cabinet's current certification.

2001.3 – The biosafety cabinet air flow ("Magnehelic") gauge should be checked (reading is equal to approximately 0.5 inches) to assure proper operation of the cabinet before placing any materials into it. Readings indicate relative pressure drop across the HEPA filter. Higher readings may, therefore, indicate filter clogging. Zero readings may indicate loss of filter integrity. In either of these cases, notify the Laboratory BSO or Laboratory Director immediately and do NOT use the hood until the problem is corrected.

2001.4 – NEVER place anything over the front or rear grille of a biosafety cabinet.

2001.5 – Disrupting the airflow into the front grille allows contaminated air from inside the cabinet to blow into the lab or directly at the person sitting at the cabinet. It also allows non-sterile air from the room to blow into the biosafety cabinet over the specimens.

2001.6 – Materials should be placed in the cabinet so as not to block air flow into the rear grille. Leave a few inches for air to flow around objects. Any disruption of the air flow in the cabinet decreases its effectiveness.

2001.7 – Before manipulating infectious materials, make sure that you have everything you need in the cabinet. The fewer times you pull your hands out of the cabinet, the less disruption of the air flow.

2001.8 – Work should be performed in the center of the work surface of the cabinet whenever possible. Work outward progressing from clean to dirty (contaminated). However, infectious agents should not be placed directly adjacent to or directly on the intake grilles.

2001.9 – After manipulating infectious agents, make sure all containers are tightly closed.

2001.10 – All waste generated by work in the cabinet should be disposed in red trash bags or sharps containers. Never put this waste in the uncontaminated white bag trash cans.

2001.11 – After the cabinet has been emptied, wipe interior surfaces with 10% bleach, followed by 70% alcohol. Wait at least 10 minutes before shutting down the BSC's fans.

NOTE: Though Class IIB cabinets are hard-ducted (so that all air is removed from the room), Class IIA cabinets recirculate about 70% of the air inside themselves and exhaust the remainder to the lab. Any use of volatile solvents, such as absolute ethanol, should be kept to a minimum or done elsewhere. Dangerously high levels of volatile vapors can accumulate inside the cabinet and pose a threat of fire or explosion.

2002 – Incubators

2002.1 – Upright Incubators

A. Incubators are normally set at 37°C.

B. Temperature should be checked each day by all users.

C. Operation manuals are located in the microbiology lab.

D. If an alarm is sounding, check the panel to identify the blinking light.
    1. If there is no obvious reason for the alarm, contact the Lab BSO or Lab Director.
    2. The "CO2 Low" (or High) message indicates a deviation from 5% CO_2. Check the hose from the wall to the unit.
    3. The "tank farm" must be checked for empty CO_2 tanks once per week.

E. Decontaminate incubators at least every week.

2003 – Autoclave
    (See Appendix A)

2004 – Emergency Equipment

2004.1 – Fire Extinguisher, located at the end of laboratory.

A. Operation

1. Fire extinguishers should be used only if the fire is small and confined to one small area Use judgment on this. Do not create a life-threatening situation while trying to extinguish a fire. If the fire is too large to put out with a fire extinguisher, evacuate the lab and activate the hospital's emergency fire response.

2. To operate the fire extinguisher, pull the pin to release the handle.

3. Stand at a safe distance from the fire (as directed on the fire extinguisher).

4. Aim the nozzle at the base of the fire, squeeze the handle to discharge the agent, and sweep completely left and right until a few seconds after seeing no fire.

B. Maintenance

Fire extinguishers are inspected annually by Maintenance. Check the gauge periodically to ensure operational status. Call Maintenance at extension XXXX if you have any questions.

2004.2 – Telephones are located at each section of the lab.

2005 – Repair and Service

Lab will notify Biomed or maintenance of any broken equipment.

C. 3000 – Operational Procedures

3001 – Inventory Control System

The laboratory section supervisors are responsible for maintaining inventory.

3002 – Working inside the Biosafety Cabinet
(See Microbiology Manual)

3003 – Working outside the Biosafety Cabinet

Working outside the BSC includes such actions as transporting samples from the BSC to an incubator or other equipment.

3003.1 – Vials or tubes being transported to the centrifuge, water bath, etc. should be in a stable rack.

3003.2 – No liquid should be allowed into any drain connected to the sanitary sewer system (e.g. from a sink) unless first autoclaved.

3004 – Removing items from the Biosafety Cabinet

Sharps are disposed in the sharps container. All non-sharp solid waste is disposed in red biohazard bags. Liquid waste may be disposed down the drain after autoclaving.

3005 – Internal Decontamination of the Biosafety Cabinet
(See Microbiology Manual)

3006 – Maintenance of Laboratory
(See General Laboratory Manual and SOP's)

D. 4000 – Safety Checks and Emergency Procedures

4001 – Training and Orientation

4001.1   All employees will attend training on Biosafety, Lab Safety, Infection Control, HIPAA, Fire Safety and Fire Prevention (also Radiation Safety if applicable) on employment and annual refreshers.

4002 – Personal Protective Equipment

4002.1 Personal Protective Equipment is required when working with potentially contaminated specimens. When using a biological safety cabinet, protective clothing, including gloves and a long-sleeved body covering (gown, laboratory coat, smock, coverall, or similar garment) should be worn so that hands and arms are completely covered to prevent contamination of cultures, skin and street clothing.

4002.2 Eye protection should be worn when handling infectious organisms or chemicals.

4002.3 These requirements also apply to anyone working in the area while someone else is working at the biosafety cabinet.

4003 – Waste Removal from the Lab

Housekeeping will collect the red biohazard bags, white (uncontaminated) trash bags and sharps containers from laboratory and dispose of them.

4004 – Management of Spills

Open the Biosafety Spill Kit and drop the disinfectant absorbent pads onto the spill. If no spill kit is available, apply paper towels to absorb the spill, and then soak paper towels with 10% bleach. For spills outside the biosafety cabinet, alert others in the area. Use N95 respirator mask if there is a possibility of harmful aerosols.

Notify the Lab BSO if there has been an exposure to harmful aerosols.

4005 – Management of Accidental Exposures

In the event of an exposure to an infectious agent or material:

Intact skin
- Remove contaminated clothing.
- Vigorously wash contaminated skin for 1 minute with soap and water. There is an emergency shower at the rear of laboratory. If necessary use the emergency shower.
- Inform Employee Health and seek medical attention at the Emergency Department.

Broken, cut, or damaged skin or puncture wound
- Remove contaminated clothing.
- Vigorously wash contaminated skin for 5 minutes with soap and water. There is an emergency shower at the rear of laboratory. If necessary use the emergency shower.
- Inform Employee Health and seek medical attention at the Emergency Department, or call 911 for assistance. If you are contaminated with infectious organisms, notify the emergency responders of the contamination.

Eye
- Immediately flush eyes for at least 15 minutes with water, using an eyewash in laboratory;
- Hold eyelids away from your eyeball and rotate your eyes so that all surfaces may be washed thoroughly; and
- Inform Employee Health and seek medical attention at the Emergency Department, or call 911 for assistance. If you are contaminated with infectious organisms, notify the emergency responders of the contamination.

Ingestion or Inhalation
- Inform Employee Health and seek medical attention at the Emergency Department. or call 911 for assistance. If you are contaminated with infectious organisms, notify the emergency responders of the contamination.
- Do not induce vomiting unless advised to do so by a health care provider.

100

4006 – Medical Surveillance
>(See Annual Employee Health Screening in the Lab's Procedure Manual.)

4007 – Emergency Phone Numbers and Procedures

4007.1 Emergency Phone Numbers

Fire and Medical Emergencies 911
Police   911
Hospital Chief Executive Officer _____
Emergency Preparedness Director _____
Hospital Administrator _____
Laboratory Director _____
Laboratory BSO   _____
Hospital All Hazards Responder _____
Hospital Facility Manager _____

4007.2 Emergency Procedures
 In responding to an emergency situation, all persons must be aware of these basic concerns:

Emergency Equipment:

TELEPHONES are located in all areas of laboratory.
FIRE EXTINGUISHER is located in the rear of laboratory.
EMERGENCY EYEWASH stations are located in each section of laboratory.
EMERGENCY SHOWER is located in the rear of laboratory.

Order of Priority in an Emergency:

I. SAFETY FOR THE EMPLOYEE/STUDENT(S) IN THE LABORATORY.

1. Notify anyone else present in the lab.
2. Safety for persons in the lab must be the first consideration. The circumstances of the emergency will determine the feasibility of carrying out site control.

II. DANGER OF OUTSIDE CONTAMINATION (Site Control):
1. Do not exit building wearing contaminated clothing or protective outerwear (gown, gloves).
2. Leave biosafety cabinet on.
3. Place covers on open containers of viable agents.

4007.3 Responding to Specific Emergencies
>(See Emergency Disaster Preparedness Plan)

E. 5000 – Outside Operations

5001 – Packaging and Labeling for Shipment to Other Institutions
(See lab policies for IATA shipping)

5002 – Record keeping in Laboratory
(See General Laboratory Policy)

F. 6000 - Security
(See Security Policy)

III. Protocols
(See Laboratory Staff Responsibilities policy)

IV. Safety Manuals

1. Biosafety in Microbiological and Biomedical Laboratories, CDC-NIH, 5th edition.

2. Microbiology manuals

3. Laboratory manuals

REVIEWED AND APPROVED BY:

Philip A. Dauterman, M.D.

_____   _____01/14/2019_____
Dr. Philip Dauterman, MD, Lab Director and   Date
Acting in the Lab Biosafety Officer position

_____   _____
Infection Control Coordinator   Date

_____   _____
Emergency Preparedness Director   Date

_____   _____
Hospital Administrator   Date

_____   _____
Hospital CEO   Date

Annual reviews
(Date and Initial)

_____
_____
_____

APPENDICES

Appendix A. Autoclave procedure

Standard Operating Procedure for Safe Autoclave Operations

The purpose of this document is to provide standard operating procedures for the safe use of autoclaves. Autoclaving is a process used to destroy microorganisms and decontaminate biohazardous waste and microbiological equipment used at biosafety levels 1, 2, 3 and 4.

HAZARDS

1. Heat burns from hot materials and autoclave chamber walls and door.
2. Steam burns from residual steam coming out from autoclave and materials on completion of cycle.
3. Hot fluid scalds from boiling liquids and spillage in autoclave.
4. Hand and arm injuries when closing the door.
5. Body injury if there is an explosion.

SAFETY

To ensure the health and safety of personnel using the autoclave, it is important for each department to maintain autoclaves and to train personnel in their proper use.

1. The name of the person responsible for the autoclave shall be posted near the autoclave. This SOP should be posted on the outside of the autoclave.
2. It is the supervisor's responsibility to ensure employees are trained before operating any autoclave unit.
3. Procedural and instructional documents provided by the manufacturer must be followed.
4. Personal protective clothing and equipment must be worn when loading and unloading the autoclave.
5. Autoclaves must be inspected at least annually. Inspection is by the autoclave manufacturer's preventative maintenance contract. A basic visual inspection should be performed monthly by the person responsible for the autoclave. The inspection, service and repair records should be available upon request.
6. Biologic, chemical and mechanical indicators of sterilization may be used to validate the autoclave's effectiveness.

PERSONAL PROTECTIVE EQUIPMENT

Equipment to protect against scalds and burns include:

a)   Heat-insulating gloves that provide complete coverage of hands and forearm
b)   Lab coat
c)   Eye protection
d)   Closed-toe footwear

104

OPERATOR INSTRUCTIONS

Training

All personnel who use autoclaves must have successfully completed a training session from their supervisor on the safe operating procedures. This requirement applies to both new and experienced personnel.

Material Preparation

1. Ensure that the material is safe for autoclaving:

    a) Samples containing solvents or substances that may emit toxic fumes should not be autoclaved.
    b) Do not autoclave bleach!

2. Glassware must be inspected for cracks prior to autoclaving.

3. Prepare and package material suitably:

    a) Loose dry materials must be wrapped or bagged in steam-penetrating paper or loosely covered with aluminum foil. Wrapping too tightly will impede steam penetration, decreasing effectiveness of the process.
    b) Loosen all lids to prevent pressure buildup. All containers must be covered by a loosened lid or steam-penetrating paper.
    c) Containers of liquid must not exceed two-thirds (2/3) full, with lids loosened.
    d) Glassware must be heat-resistant borosilicate.
    e) Plastics must be heat-resistant, i.e., polycarbonate (PC), PTFE ("Teflon") and most polypropylene (PP) items.
    f) Discarded sharps must be in a designated 'Sharps' container.
    g) All items must be tagged with autoclave tape.

4. Place items in secondary containers to secure and contain spills:

    a) Items should be placed in a stainless steel pan or other autoclavable container for their stability and ease of handling.
    b) Place containers of liquid, bags of agar plates, or other materials that may boil over or leak, into a secondary pan in the autoclave.
    c) The pan must be large enough to contain a total spill of the contents.
    d) Bags must not be tightly sealed as steam cannot penetrate.

5. After autoclaving, waste liquids can be poured down the drain. Autoclaved waste solids are disposed in red trash bags.

Appendix B. Floor Diagram

LABORATORY EMERGENCY EVACUATION ROUTE

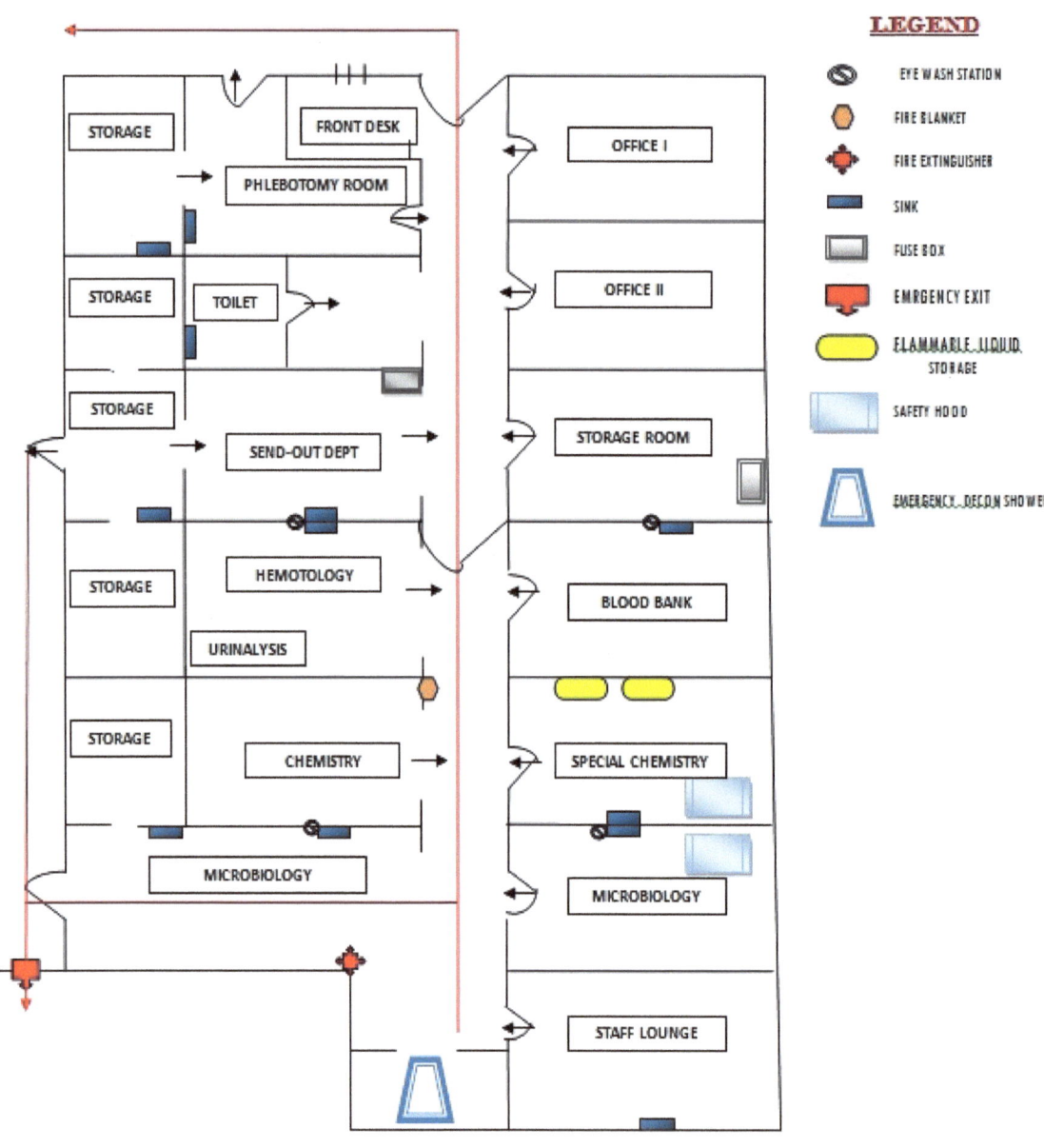

Chapter 21 – How to prepare reports for the hospital wide safety committee

An Institutional Biosafety Committee (IBC) is typically only seen in an organization with more than one biosafety officer. Hence, an IBC is commonly seen in a research institution or teaching hospital, but is not commonly seen in a small community hospital. The IBC is charged with developing institution-wide biosafety policies and procedures. The IBC also reviews research protocols and risk assessments, creation of new safety policies and settles disputes over safety matters between the various biosafety officers on the committee. If any dispute is particular contentious or sensitive the IBC will typically ask for outside advice from experts in the field. The IBC is typically composed of all the biosafety officers in the organization, representatives of the lab staff and lab management, the Lab Director and at least one representative of the Medical Staff.

Small community hospitals do not typically have an IBC. Instead the hospital-wide safety is delegated to a hospital standing committee such as the Infection Control Committee, Quality Council, Morbidity and Mortality Committee or other committee. Hospital-wide safety is mandated by the hospital's regulators and every hospital must have a committee that deals with hospital-wide safety. Regardless of which committee this is delegated to, the committee must review the accidents, exposures, incidents, etc. occurring in lab.

The membership of the hospital-wide safety committee will be stipulated in the hospital bylaws. For the Infection Control Committee this is typically the Infection Control Nurse, all Infectious Disease physicians, the hospital Risk Manager, hospital Quality Coordinator, etc. The typical hospital's bylaws do not mention the Lab BSO position. In this situation, you should ask the chair of the hospital-wide safety committee to add you as a member.

You as Lab BSO will need to prepare annual reports and submit these to the committee that oversees safety at your hospital. If there is a particularly bad occurrence you will likely be asked to prepare a report sooner than annually.

The annual report should summarize staff turnover and document that all new incoming staff have had appropriate training in lab biosafety, PPE, infection control, etc. The annual report should discuss any changes in facilities and document that old facilities and equipment were properly disinfected before being decommissioned and disposed of, all new facilities were properly designed and all new equipment meets specifications. All incidents and other significant events occurring during the year should be summarized. An example report is given on the following page.

MY LABORATORY
123 My Street
My Town, XY 98765

MEMORANDUM

To: Institutional Biosafety Committee

From: Dr. Philip Dauterman, Laboratory Director and Biosafety Officer   *Philip A. Dauterman, MD* _____

Date: January 14, 2019

Subject: Annual Laboratory Biosafety Officer report for 2018

Thank you for giving me the opportunity to summarize the events of 2018. During the course of 2018 two staff members resigned as they were relocating out of state. Two new staff were hired to fill the vacancies. The newly hired staff include phlebotomist John Doe hired in April and lab technologist Jane Doe hired in September. In my capacity as Lab Biosafety Officer I oversaw their orientation and competency testing in all aspects of lab safety. The newly hired staff demonstrated more than adequate competency and I signed their competency testing documentation without reservations.

The only new equipment acquired during the year was lab's new autoclave, installed in November. Lab's new autoclave meets all specifications for sterilization. It passed validated using autoclave tape, mechanical and biologic indicators of sterilization. The first trial run of the autoclave was unsuccessful with melting of the autoclave trash bag and dripping of liquefied agar throughout the inside of the autoclave. It took housekeeping more than an hour to clean out the mess on the inside of the autoclave. This problem was remediated by setting the autoclave to a lower temperature setting and placing a metal pan under the autoclave bag. The problem of melting autoclave bags did not recur.

Only one accident occurred in laboratory in 2018. In April there was a spill of less than 100ml of 10% formalin in the histology section. The Root Cause Analysis determined that this was due to ill-fitting formalin container lids. All unused defective formalin containers were returned to the vendor in exchange for containers with properly fitted lids. The hospital's procurement office was asked to change vendors for the next order of formalin containers. So far there has been no recurrence of ill-fitting formalin container lids.

In summary, 2018 was a relatively uneventful year. There were no other incidents reported and no changes in staff, equipment or facilities in addition to those described above.

Chapter 22 – Lab Biosafety Officer qualifications, hiring, retention and competency assessment

Laboratory Biosafety Officer (BSO) positions largely did not exist prior to the 1990s. The lab biosafety work was distributed among the lab staff, lab supervisor, and lab director. Following the anthrax mailings in 2001, laboratory biosafety and biosecurity became much more of a concern nationwide. The Centers for Disease Control and Prevention (CDCP) funded numerous Lab BSO positions at public health labs nationwide beginning about the time of the Ebola outbreak in 2014.

Lab BSO positions are new. There is no formal degree for these positions. No universities anywhere are offering a degree in Lab Biosafety Officer. The American Biological Safety Association (ABSA) is offering registration and certification as a Biosafety Professional.

The typical minimum qualifications for hiring as a Lab BSO include:

1. Earned bachelor's, masters or doctoral level degree in microbiology, medical technology, or related sciences.
2. At least two years work experience in a laboratory.
3. Knowledge of BSL-2 (and if applicable BSL-2+, BSL-3 and BSL-4) equipment and practices.
4. Must pass appropriate background checks (police clearance).

Hiring a Lab BSO has been very difficult. The lab where I work created the position in 2014 but the position was vacant for nearly a year before someone could be hired into the position. The former Lab BSO stayed in the position for about 2 years, vacating the position in September, 2017. A replacement could not be found in the short term and I was appointed as "acting" in the position until someone else could be found to fill the position on a permanent basis.

In terms of staffing, the Lab BSO position is not considered essential at most small hospital labs. At the lab where I work, the position did not exist prior to 2014. The position was not filled until the next year due to a lack of applicants. Prior to filling the lab BSO position, the lab biosafety work was distributed among the lab staff, lab supervisor and lab director. The Lab BSO position is not mentioned in the CLIA regulations governing clinical laboratories. Thus, there was never any regulatory requirement for this position to be filled. The Lab BSO position may be considered more essential in large microbiology and public health labs as these types of labs would deal with more serious infectious pathogens.

In my experience retention of a Lab BSO has been impossible. When the former Lab BSO resigned I offered him higher salary to stay on. He refused saying that he was leaving for other reasons. He has young children and couldn't handle being on-call 24 hours a day 7 days a week. He left for a less stressful administrative job. After he left I was assigned the added duties of the Lab BSO position in addition to my Lab Director position. I would like to hand off the Lab BSO duties to the next person, but no one is coming in the near term. That is part of the reason I am writing this book - so it can be the orientation for the next person to take the Lab BSO position.

In the typical hospital the Lab Director is the immediate supervisor to the Lab BSO. The Lab BSO is supervisory to all the lab staff except possibly the Lab Supervisor. You as Lab BSO should review the chain of command and organizational chart at your hospital to determine if you are supervisory, equal or subordinate to the Lab Supervisor position. In any event you will typically be subordinate to the Lab Director position. In my case I am both the Lab Director and Lab BSO at the same time so I am subordinate to the Hospital's Medical Director and Hospital Administrator and supervisory to everyone in lab.

If you are assuming an existing Lab BSO position you should ask for at least a one to two month orientation from the departing Lab BSO with handover of all documents. If you are assuming a newly created Lab BSO position you will not likely receive much orientation as no one has occupied your Lab BSO position before. In my case, the departing Lab BSO quit on short notice. I was familiar with the work the departed Lab BSO was doing, and was able to figure everything out from the paperwork left behind by the departed Lab BSO.

In terms of promotion and career advancement, the next higher positions in lab are the Lab Supervisor and Lab Director positions. In my experience the turnover of these positions is very slow, such that you may be waiting many years if you are looking for internal promotion. Furthermore, the qualifications of the Lab Director position largely preclude anyone other than a pathologist from occupying the position. Most Lab BSO departures I have seen have been lateral transfers. For example the Lab BSO who quit from my lab took a Materials Countermeasures (i.e. chemical hazard preparedness) position which was essentially a lateral transfer to a different government agency.

The competency testing of the Lab BSO should encompass all aspects of the Lab BSO position. As with all competency assessment in lab, there is typically a form used for this purpose. In some labs there is a specific form used for Lab BSO competency evaluation, In other labs a general lab competency evaluation form or a hospital-wide competency evaluation form is used.

The typical lab evaluation form has checkboxes for "Pass", "Fail" or "Not applicable". This is to meet regulatory requirements for lab tech competency testing. Your Lab BSO competency evaluation paperwork will probably have the same checkboxes as it is likely to be made from the same template used for lab tech competency testing. I have seen other rating systems, with the checkboxes labeled "Entry Level", "Midlevel" and "Senior Level".

Most but not all hospital competency testing forms have an overall grade, such as "Pass" or "Fail". Another possibility is overall grades of "Outstanding", "Satisfactory", "Marginal" and "Fail".

For a lab tech, it is a regulatory requirement to pass competency testing. If any line on a lab tech's competency testing form is marked as a "Fail" it must be remediated before he or she can continue with the patient testing. There is no such regulatory requirement for the Lab BSO position. From a regulatory standpoint, nothing would stop you from continuing to work after a failed competency testing. However, the Human Resources (HR) department of your hospital would probably require you to have retraining, retake the competency assessment and pass it in order to keep your job.

As with all competency testing, the evaluation form is filled out behind closed doors. You will typically be called for a closed door meeting with your immediate supervisor and presented with the findings. You will be asked to sign the competency testing form. There is typically a field on the form for you to write in any responses if you want. The form is typically filed in a folder kept in a locked file cabinet in lab with a copy going to the hospital's HR department.

I will give an example of a Lab BSO competency testing form on the next page.

Title	*Position*	*Type of Evaluation*	*Employee Name:*
Training and Competency Checklist	Laboratory Biosafety Officer	☐ Initial Training ☐ Annual Competency ☐ Other:_____	Position Title:_____ Date of Hire: _____ Date of Assignment:_____

See Page 2 For Instructions to Complete Form

	Policy, Procedure, Function	Y	N	N/A
	LABORATORY BIOSAFETY OFFICER			
1	Able to list the various classes of lab hazards and distinguish hazardous items from items that are not hazardous.			
2	Able to list and describe the PPE needed to handle chemical and biologic hazards in lab.			
3	Able to describe the PPE needed for each task in laboratory. Able to demonstrate proper donning and doffing of all PPE used in laboratory.			
4	Able to explain all relevant safety signage and labeling needed for chemical and biologic hazards.			
5	Able to describe the routes of exposure associated with Laboratory Acquired Infections (LAI).			
6	Able to describe procedures designed to minimize the risk of LAI.			
7	Able to identify which infectious agents require BSL-2, BSL-3 or BSL-4 containment from a list of the commonly tested organisms at this lab.			
8	Able to identify the PPE and practices needed for BSL-2, BSL-3 and BSL-4.			
9	Able to describe storage and handling procedures for cultures of organisms.			
10	Able to name the most commonly used hazardous materials chemicals in the lab.			
11	Able to interpret the information on a Safety Data Sheet (SDS).			
12	Able to identify the PPE and practices needed for handling the lab's hazardous chemicals (acids, corrosives, flammables, etc.).			
13	Able to describe storage and handling procedures for hazardous materials chemicals.			
14	Able to develop response plans for disasters, chemical spills and/or accidental release of cultured organisms. Able to write policies, procedures and a Biosafety Manual. Able to prepare reports.			
15	Able to describe the proper disposal of waste including sharps, solid and liquid waste contaminated with chemical or biological hazard.			
16	Able to describe the physical hazards in lab and the procedures used to minimize the physical hazard risks in lab.			
17	Able to describe lab's security including door locks, visitor policy and restrictions on visitors.			
18	Able to list the lab's disinfection and sterilization methods.			
19	Able to describe proper use of the autoclave including biologic, chemical and mechanical indicators of sterilization.			
20	Able to describe all relevant regulations regarding lab's chemical, biological and physical hazards.			
21	Able to describe lab's incident reporting system.			
22	The Lab BSO adheres to all lab safety polices and has attended all required trainings, complies with the hospital's Employee Health program, is not delinquent for annual health clearance, has appropriate leadership and communication skills and enforces safety on the lab staff.			
	OTHER NOT LISTED ABOVE:			

Comments:

_____

_____

Employee Signature:_____   Date:_____

Supervisor Signature:_____   Date:_____

Lab Director Signature:_____   Date:_____

INITIAL TRAINING AND COMPETENCY CHECKLIST LABORATORY BIOSAFETY OFFICER

Instructions for Supervisor/Evaluator

- Refer to competency testing policy for general information.
- Use the following symbols to indicate competence:

Y: Yes, competent

N: No, needs training

N/A: Item not applicable

- If any failure to demonstrate competence is observed, the evaluator must initiate and complete a "Competency: Remediation Form". See the competency remediation procedure.
- Have employee sign and date the evaluation form indicating that he/she agrees with the evaluation.

Instructions for Employee

If you feel that the training and competency evaluation is inadequate or inappropriate, ask for a conference to include the Lab Supervisor and Lab Director.

INDEX

Pictures of me having a bad year in 2015

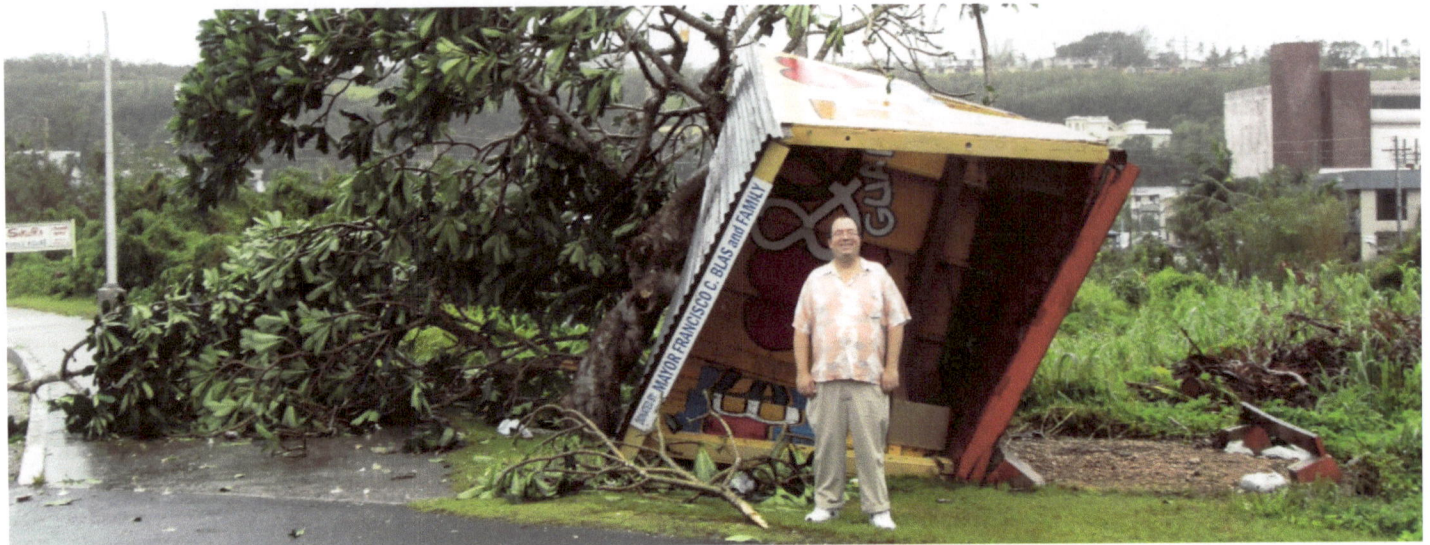

Picture of me on Guam the day after Typhoon Dolphin. I was on a temporary 2 week assignment to Guam in May, 2015 when Typhoon Dolphin hit. This photo shows typical Category 1 Hurricane damage – flimsy wooden structure overturned but not completely disintegrated. The tree trunk is still standing with large branches down on the sidewalk. There is no damage to any concrete structure in this photo.

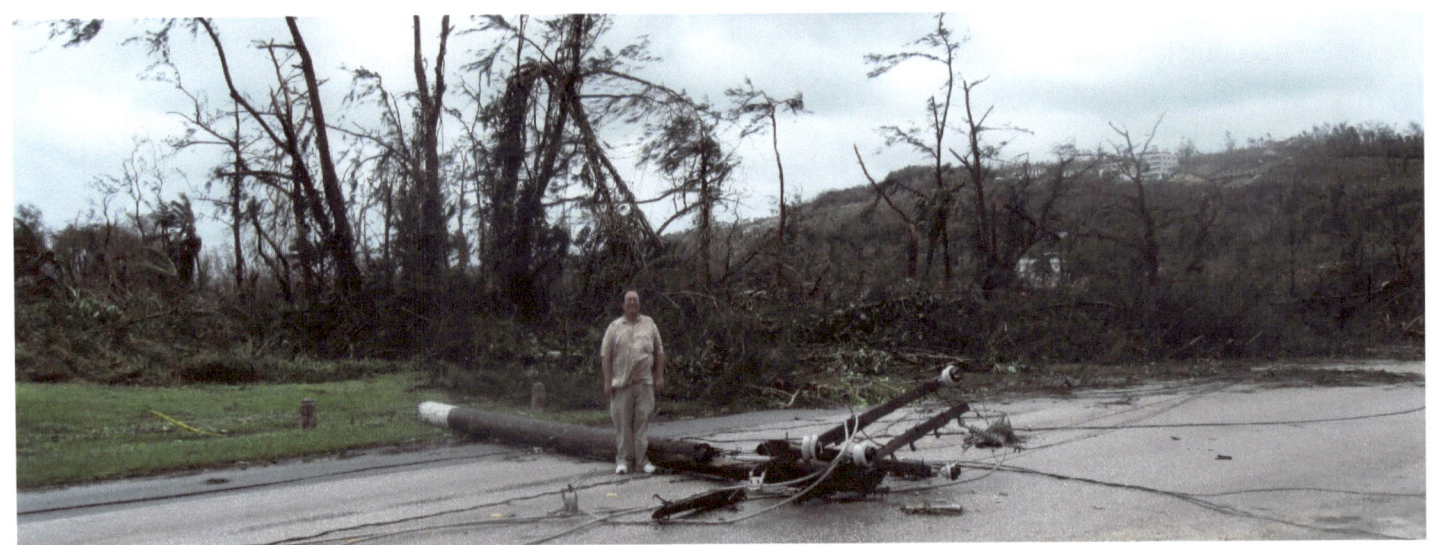

Picture of me on Saipan the day after Typhoon Soudelor. I work full time on Saipan where Typhoon Soudelor hit August 2, 2015. This photo shows hurricane damage typical of Category 3 or higher – a downed telephone pole with multiple large trees broken at the trunk or entirely uprooted. An entire forest has been felled, such that structures are visible on the distant hillside that would not ordinarily be visible through a forest. Disintegrated structures and debris from disintegrated structures can be seen on the hillside.

I lost 23 pounds on the Hurricane Diet Plan

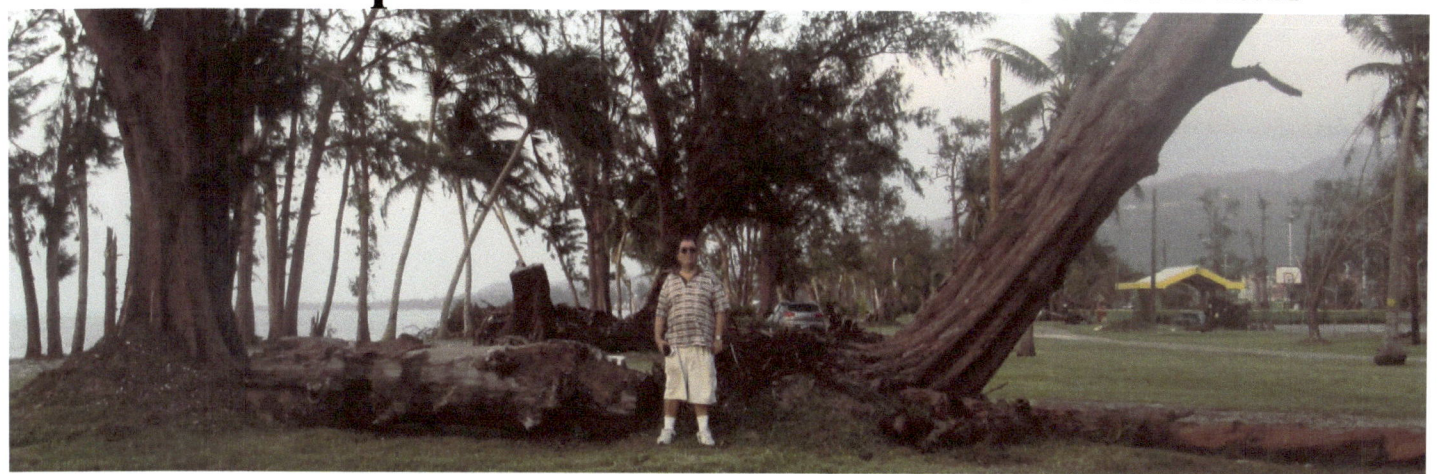

Picture of me on Saipan taken October 24, 2015 about two and a half months after Typhoon Soudelor hit August 2. The debris has been largely removed but a few downed trees remain. In the background, both concrete and wooden phone poles can be seen. Each concrete phone pole replaces a downed wooden phone pole. At the time of this photo, my apartment still did not have electric power restored after the storm. In that time I lost 23 pounds, down from 248 pounds at the time of the storm to 225 pounds in this photo. If you don't have electric power you can't cook your food and your refrigerator doesn't work either. After a major hurricane, the food supply will be so disrupted you literally won't know where your next meal is coming from. I refer to this as the Hurricane Diet Plan.

About the author

Dr. Dauterman received his M.D. Degree from Ross University followed by residency training in anatomical and clinical pathology at Eastern Virginia Medical School in Norfolk, Virginia. He completed his pathology training with a surgical pathology fellowship at SUNY Health Science Center, Brooklyn, New York. He spent the next 16 years practicing pathology at Guam Memorial Hospital, initially as a staff pathologist and eventually Laboratory Director. During his time on Guam, he served as a pathology consultant for the U.S. Navy. Dr. Dauterman accepted a Pathologist position at Jack C. Montgomery VAMC, Muskogee, OK for one year.

Dr. Dauterman returned to the Mariana Islands where he is currently serving as a Laboratory Director and Consultant for Saipan and provides consultation as needed to public health departments in the US affiliated pacific islands.

Dr. Dauterman is board certified in Anatomic and Clinical Pathology and a Fellow of the College of American Pathologists.

This book is a practical guide designed for physicians, medical technologists and scientists involved in Laboratory Medicine. Pathologists and pathology residents may find it especially useful as these topics are rarely covered in-depth during the rigorous training of pathology. Dr. Dauterman's practical advice covers all hazards including biological, chemical and physical hazards.

About the Author is written by Timothy Sorrells, MD

www.ingramcontent.com/pod-product-compliance
Lightning Source LLC
Chambersburg PA
CBHW050849180526
45159CB00007B/2624